Guns and Bandages

A Combat Medic in Israel's Army, 1961-1978

David J. Mendelsohn

Pippin Publishing

Copyright © 2003 by Pippin Publishing Corporation
Suite 232, 85 Ellesmere Road
Toronto, Ontario
Canada M1R 4B9

All rights reserved. No part of this publication may be reproduced or transmitted in any form or by any means, electronic, mechanical, or otherwise, including photocopying and recording, or sotred in any retrieval system without express permission in writing from the publisher.

Designed by John Zehethofer
Typeset by Jay Tee Graphics Ltd.
Maps drawn by Christopher Johnson
Printed and bound in Canada by AGMV Marquis Imprimeur Inc.

We acknowledge the financial support of the Government of Canada through the Book Industry Development Program for our publishing activities.
We acknowledge the support of the Government of Ontario through the Ontario Media Development Corporation's Ontario Book Initiative.

National Library of Canada Cataloguing in Publication

Mendelsohn, David

    Guns and bandages : a combat medic in Israel's army, 1961-1978 / David J. Mendelsohn.
ISBN 0-88751-101-5

    1. Mendelsohn, David. 2. Medicine, Military—Israel. 3. Israel—Armed Forces—Medical personnel—Biography. I. Title.

H347.M45A3 2003   355.3'45'092   C2003-900754-5

10 9 8 7 6 5 4 3 2 1

To Dudu – superb leader, soldier, gentleman and gentle man – this book is affectionately dedicated.

Acknowledgements

The melody and the Hebrew lyrics of *Yerushalayim Shel Zahav (Jerusalem of Gold)* were composed by Naomi Shemer and published by Chappell/Warner Publishers. Her lyrics are reproduced here with her kind permission. The sensitive and evocative translation of the lyrics into English was beautifully made by Chaya Galai, who has graciously given me permission to use them in my book.

I acknowledge the love and support of my family throughout my writing of this memoir: my wife, Jenny, my children Lee and Roberto, Noa and Dan, and Jonathan, and my grandchildren Simon and Gabriel.

David Mendelsohn

Toronto
August, 2003

Table of Contents

"Chovesh!" .... page 9

Part I: 1961–June, 1967 .... page 11

Part II: The Six Day War .... page 73

Part III: Between the Six Day War and The Outbreak
            of the Yom Kippur War .... page 115

Page IV: The Yom Kippur War .... page 139

Part V: From Ismailia to Toronto .... page 193

Epilog: .... page 203

List of Illustrations and Maps

At a picnic for South African immigrants to Israel, Ben Shemen Forest, 1961. I am sitting in the front row, looking pensive ....page 39
Returning from a route march during basic training. Surprisingly, after such a gruelling march, I look quite spry ....page 43
Some of the South Africans at the completion of basic training. I am in the front row, second from left, and next to me is a (balding) Ivan ....page 52
At the Church of the Nativity, Bethlehem, with my platoon commander, Yossie; June, 1967 ....page 97
Jenny "disguised" as a soldier, touring the West Bank, June 1967 ....page 110
Yitzchak Rabin, our Commander-in-Chief, reviewing us as we marched past in the Victory Parade ....page 112
Victory Parade of the Jerusalem Brigade, held at Givat Ram shortly after the Six Day War. The rifles support helmets, each of which contains a flame representing one of the fallen ....page 112
Guarding in a *mutzav* on the banks of the Jordan River, 1969 ....page 120
At the Sweetwater Canal, October, 1973 ....page 156
With two U.N. peacekeepers near Ismailia, late 1973 ....page 163
Preparing to edit the two doctors' articles in the middle of the desert. They (seated left) look happy and confident, but I (standing) look decidedly apprehensive ....page 166

Illustrations and Maps (continued)

The demob pin-up calendar. Early 1974..................................page 182
Cooking *luf* to while away the time while waiting in the
    desert for our wives' arrival...page 184
Jenny and I standing on the military road built by the Israeli
    army across the Suez Canal. With the eventual reopening
    of the Suez Canal, the road was demolished ....page 185
Breakfast near Ismailia for our visiting wives. Jenny is in a
    striped top, sitting at our improvised table ....page 188
Dudu, my beloved commandeer, to whom I have dedicated
    this book. Jerusalem, 2002..page 206
War memorial to the soldiers who fell in the battle for the
    U.N. Headquarters in June, 1967...page 208
The photograph on the outside back cover is of David at the
    time of his arrival in Israel and enlistment in the Nachal
    Regiment.

List of Maps

Israel in June, 1961 ....page 12
Jerusalem on the Eve of the Six Day War: June 5, 1967 ....page 74
The Suez Front, Yom Kippur War, October 1973.........................page 140

"Chovesh!"

It was a frantic cry for help

"*Chovesh*!" ("medic!") It came from about ten feet away. I scrambled over to see what had happened, bursting through a circle of about eight soldiers crouched around Shimon, who lay sprawled on the hard earth. They were all in a state bordering on panic and, to make matters worse, Jordanian mortar shells continued to crash around us. Shimon and I had served together in this infantry platoon for several years and I knew him fairly well: a very quiet, decent man, of whom everyone was fond. Like me, he was a private. He was an immigrant from North Africa and had been in Israel for, I would reckon, some ten to fifteen years. Each of the soldiers surrounding him had, in their panic, taken out the single sterile bandage that every man carries and opened the packaging, thereby rendering them non-sterile and useless.

Shimon was lying in the middle of the circle, unconscious, with a faint trickle of blood dribbling down his face from where a piece of shrapnel had grazed his head. The soldiers all began shouting at me to dress this wound. But we had been taught that, before you begin dressing visible wounds, you must first examine the soldier to see if there are any concealed wounds that may be more serious. I ripped open Shimon's shirt, and there it was: a large piece of shrapnel, with hideously jagged edges, lodged deep in his chest. I followed regulations and dressed the wound, but I knew that Shimon was already dead.

That was June 5, 1967, the first day of the Six Day War, and that was the day that I first saw combat and was forced to put my medical training to the test.

PART I

1961 – JUNE, 1967

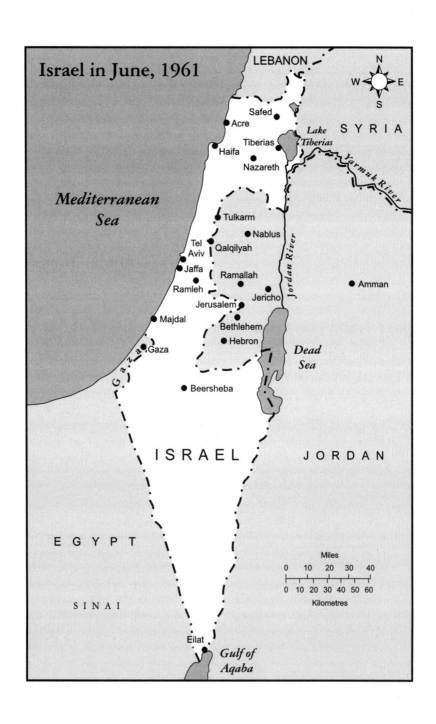

Like Shimon I was born in Africa, but in South Africa, in Johannesburg in 1944, so that to all intents and purposes I was a post World War Two baby. And my birth, in as remote a land as South Africa where my family had immigrated in the first decade of the twentieth century, protected me from the horrors of war and Holocaust.

My parents were typical South African Jews of that generation, both being born there to immigrant parents, my father Maurice in 1910, and my mother, Hilary, in 1914. My father's parents came to South Africa from Lithuania after the terrible pogroms that were part of Jewish life in the Czar's empire. As is so common with waves of immigration, once the first Lithuanian Jews had arrived it did not take long before they saved up and sent for relatives; word spread, and more and more followed. Most South African Jews have their roots in Lithuania, with a sizable minority coming from Great Britain and Germany. Although my paternal grandparents' first language was Yiddish, my father and his siblings never became fluent speakers of Yiddish, although they clearly understood it.

My mother's parents came to South Africa from Great Britain. I only have sketchy information, but as far as I have been able to ascertain my grandparents were first or second generation British, their parents having come originally from either Central or Eastern Europe one or two generations earlier. What I do have is a copy of my maternal grandparents' birth certificates, showing that my grandmother, Elizabeth Catherine Sarah Jacobs, was born in the County of Middlesex in 1877; her mother's name was Miriam, née Berlyn, and her father's name was Julius Jacobs; his occupation is given as "commercial traveler." My grandfather, Isaac Marks, was born in Birmingham in 1878; his mother's name was Sarah, née Kristal, and his father Samuel's occupation is given as "hawker" – at that time a popular line of work with immigrants. My mother's family was staunchly Victorian in their manners and outlook and, from what she told me, there was no vestige of Yiddish in her home, although I am sure that her parents must have known the language.

Financial circumstances in my father's family determined that only one of the three siblings could go to university. His younger sister, Aunt Stella, being female was thereby automatically excluded from the running, and my grandparents evidently decided that his brother, Uncle Jack, should go because he was the "cleverer of the boys." This blocked my father from realizing his dream of becoming a lawyer. Instead he became a bookkeeper, and by 1961 had become the comptroller of a large clothing firm in Johannesburg.

My mother, too, was not able to realize her career dream of becoming a nurse because her authoritarian, Victorian, father decreed that that was not a profession "for a good Jewish girl." This she dutifully accepted, becoming instead first a shorthand typist and then, in mid-career, a successful nursery school teacher. Later, for reasons I shall make apparent, she once again became a shorthand typist, but nevertheless was to live her entire life with a deep and ever-present regret that she never became a nurse.

My parents, like most South African Jews to this day, were non-observant members of an Orthodox synagogue. That notwithstanding, my brother and I were taken to services weekly without really understanding clearly what it was all about any more than my parents did, and in our home we did not observe the rules of Kashrut or of the Sabbath.

Both my parents I would describe as apolitical. They grew up in a racist South Africa, where privilege was thrust upon them simply by virtue of their having white skin. And this way of life became even more entrenched with the rise to power in 1948 of the National Party, which coined the phrase 'Apartheid' and institutionalized racial separation in law. The National Party intensified the racist attitudes they had inherited from the British and from previous political parties, and strengthened white privilege yet further. Consequently my parents, in their heads largely sympathetic towards the blacks and their plight yet content to enjoy the benefits and advantages that Apartheid offered, took the same line that so many South African Jews took – don't rock the boat. There was always the subconscious fear of what would happen if the blacks were ever to come to power – a fear that the government had very successfully instilled in all whites. Moreover, everyone was acutely aware that the Apartheid government was a ruthless authoritarian regime, and that any attempt to oppose it was a deadly game entailing the most dire of consequences. Not only were my parents uninvolved in politics, they were also uninvolved in the vibrant Zionist movement of South African Jewry, refraining from participating in any of the Zionist organizations and remaining largely uninformed about the events unfolding in the Middle East as the State of Israel was born in 1948 and then struggled for its existence.

I have only one brother, Steve, almost three years older than me, and we grew up together in a very pleasant middle-class neighborhood in Johannesburg, where we attended government schools. A few years after we completed our schooling it became the norm for Jewish children to go to Jewish Day Schools, but in our day this was not the case, and in fact there was only one such school when I was growing up, located at the opposite end of Johannesburg from where we lived. Ours was a mixed neighborhood of Jews and non-Jews, but of course all white (by law). At our elementary school the Jews were a significant minority; at high school, which was fed by several elementary schools in the same general area, the proportion of Jews still remained fairly high.

My parents may have been untouched by Zionism, but when we were growing up Zionism was nevertheless a strong force in South Africa. The left-of-centre Zionist Youth Movement 'Habonim' ('The Builders') flourished, and my older cousins Marie and Ann, then Steve, and then I all joined the movement. Habonim began as a Jewish clone of the Boy Scouts, but had a pronounced overlay of Zionist Socialist ideals, which soon became more important than the scouting. The movement was divided into three age groups, each with an ideology related to the development and protection of Israel: The youngest, up to age twelve, were called 'shtilim' ('saplings') and the ideology was built around the planting of seeds. Then, from twelve to sixteen, there were the 'bonim' ('builders'), and they were building the State of Israel and much of the imagery was of bricks and building. Finally, the oldest group, from sixteen onwards, were the 'shomrim' ('the guards') guarding Israel.

Habonim held regular weekly meetings in each suburb, and for all the different age groups. The meetings, where boys and girls met together, were a stimulating mix of games, songs and folk dances, together with some appropriately pitched educational program usually about some aspect of Israel. For the younger age groups, of course, the focus was more on having fun than on learning about Zionism, Israel and Socialist philosophy, but the balance gradually shifted in the *bonim* group. The most attractive part of being in Habonim was the three-week summer camp by the ocean, in which in my day some 1,000 children participated, and a two-week educational seminar held at a boarding school during the winter break.

In the oldest age group, *shomrim*, Habonim called on all its members to give expression to their ideals by making Aliyah, (immigrating, or literally 'going up' to Israel), and settling on a kibbutz, a communal agricultural settlement.

As I grew in Habonim, I began to question the world around me, specifically white South African society, and began fervently to believe that the society that was being built in Israel was a more just and virtuous way for people to live.

My parents were not Zionists, so were certainly not the people who encouraged us to join Habonim – on the contrary, if anything they were a little leery of it, disapproving of the fact that the meetings for the older age group took place on Friday nights, the eve of the Sabbath. Non-observant though we were, this was always very much a family night with us, to be spent together with my Aunt Madge, Uncle Jack and cousins Marie and Ann. The trail was blazed by my two cousins who finally succeeded in persuading their parents to let them join the movement, and in due course to go to meetings on a Friday night. By the time I wanted to join, resistance from my parents had ceased. They not only allowed me to join, but did not even fight us when it came time to attend Friday night meetings, although this effectively destroyed our family night ritual. Being a Jewish organization, and knowing the importance of Friday night even for the non-observant, it might seem strange that Habonim selected that night for their meetings. The reason for this was that the younger age groups in Habonim met on Sunday mornings, and at these meetings the members in the oldest age group functioned as counselors; however they, too, needed an opportunity to enjoy a program with their peers, so since Friday nights seemed the best time from the young people's perspective, this became the night they selected.

Habonim was an extremely important part of my education during those formative years, and I will always be grateful to my counselors, to Giddy in particular, today a professor at the Hebrew University and still a dear friend. I joined around the time I began high school, and never tire of claiming that I received my real education not from the Apartheid-controlled government school I attended, but from Habonim. Whereas state-run education did not want students to think too much lest they begin to question their reality, Habonim was dedicated to making us think – and to think about such matters as equality and justice for all. Topics of this nature were subversive in South Africa at that time, and care was taken not to publicize everything we were learning. I vividly recall studying the Communist Manifesto with Giddy. This was banned literature at the time in South Africa, and the mere possession of a copy could result in imprisonment. Consequently, we were admonished never to breathe a word to our parents or indeed to anyone about what we were studying and, well aware of the danger, we all observed this without fail.

Another example of the type of education we were receiving from Habonim was epitomized by the winter seminar I attended, the theme of which was 'Freedom.' Needless to say, the ideas and ideals we were being educated towards at that seminar would not have been well received by the government of the day, since Habonim's educational program led to us reflect critically on the society in which we lived. At the winter seminar we not only spent hours discussing all the different aspects of freedom that should exist in a truly democratic state, but were also made acutely aware of the inequalities existing in our very own society, which completely lacked equality of opportunity, equality before the law, a free press, and freedom of association. As a result, I began to consider making Aliyah to Israel, where I believed a more just social order prevailed.

The people who 'graduated' from Habonim could be divided into three main groups: those who carried on with their adult lives in South Africa, largely closing their eyes to the injustice; those who made Aliyah, like Steve and me; and those who became actively involved in anti-apartheid politics. The last group was small but not insignificant, and at least two of my peers served prison terms for their activities, and were ultimately exiled from South Africa by the government. They became involved in the South African struggle largely as a result of activism on the university campuses – there students held meetings and rallies, and offered various kinds of assistance to the black members of the African National Congress. Tension between the three groups of Habonim graduates scarcely existed, because those who stayed in South Africa and shut their eyes to what was happening, and that very small group who stayed and became politically active, dropped out of the movement around the time that we finished high school.

The scouting component remained, even when we were in the oldest age group, and this guaranteed wonderful social events and summer camps under canvas. But what was much more important for me was the education in values I was receiving. We were taught about justice, democracy and the equality of all people regardless of race, color or creed. And, of course, we were taught about Israel, the fledgling Jewish state, and particularly about Labor-Socialist Zionism and its philosophy of returning to the land and of the dignity of manual labor. And most important of all, we were educated and strongly encouraged to give practical expression to our ideals by immigrating to Israel.

I was one of those who was entranced by these exciting, novel ideas. I loved the values we were being taught, was hypnotized by the magic of the birth of Israel, and was simultaneously totally convinced of the immorality of the South African regime. Habonim had become central to my whole being, providing me with a full and satisfying social life. As I think back on those days and try to understand how my parents must have felt about my intense involvement in Habonim, I realize that until confronting them with my decision to make Aliyah I seldom, if ever, actually discussed with them what it was we did at Habonim. Once I was part of the *shomrim* group, the place where we discussed Aliyah and our futures in either South Africa or Israel was not at the regular meetings, since most of my fellow Habonim members were not so determined to emigrate; instead, a special group was formed, one committed to Aliyah, and it held its own meetings. This was a group called a 'garin' ('a seed'), the aim of which was to settle together in Israel. Traditionally, a *garin* left as a group, and all settled on the same agricultural kibbutz. Our *garin* was different – we were a group of people, all university students or soon to be university students, and we wanted to set up a communal society like on a kibbutz, but located instead in a small town of immigrants, the idea being that we would live by the socialist principles of the kibbutz, but in an urban, professional setting. We were not the first to come up with this idea, nor were we the first to fail. Our *garin* was made up of people at very different stages in their studies, and although most members did make Aliyah, the communal living idea never materialized. The reason was that not only did we all arrive in Israel at different times that spanned a number of years, but our ideal was not realistic – Israel has seen numerous attempts at the creation of socialist, kibbutz-like urban settlements, and, to the best of my knowledge, they have all failed.

By my mid teens I knew that what I wanted most in the world was to settle in Israel. Realizing this goal would automatically separate me from the Apartheid regime, which I had come to hate and of which I was so bitterly ashamed to be a member. These two goals combined into an irresistible force, propelling me inexorably forwards and helping to shape my life.

Paradoxically, notwithstanding the intense and obviously successful Zionist education we received, Habonim never placed any emphasis on military service in Israel, or on educating us to the fact that if we went to live in Israel, we would be required to do national service and then 'miluim' (reserve duty) for years and years afterwards. I have thought a great deal about why this was – after all, *Tzahal* (The Israel Defense Force) and serving in the army is such a central facet of everyone's life in Israel. Immigration to Israel and successful integration into Israeli society is, I believe, inextricably entwined with *Tzahal* and military service, and yet this necessary aspect of Israeli life was always played down and barely if ever mentioned. I think that the main reason for this approach was probably that Habonim was basically anti-militaristic in its philosophy, although I do have two possible additional explanations for this omission. First, I think that if more emphasis had been placed on military service and all that this entailed, this would have discouraged some potential immigrants from going. In addition, I have come to the conclusion that this was Habonim's reaction to the more militant right-wing Zionist movement, *Betar*, which trumpeted the achievements of the Israeli army, tending to glorify it almost as an end in itself. After all the years I've lived in Israel and to this day, I see this failure to deal with the army service question as a major educational error by Habonim, since it left a number of its members ill-prepared for life in Israel and facing many difficulties successfully integrating into Israeli society.

As for my broader future, always fascinated by medicine, throughout my childhood and my high-school years I had set my heart on becoming a doctor. As an initial step I took several first-aid courses during my schooling. But then one winter, while I was attending a Habonim seminar, I confided in one of the counselors, Robin, my sincere intention to make Aliyah and settle in Israel.

"What do you plan on studying after you finish school?" he asked.

"Medicine," I replied without hesitation.

"Don't do that. If you are really serious about Aliyah, then forget becoming a doctor. Israel has too many doctors. You should study agronomy."

As of that moment, such was Habonim's influence over me, I promptly abandoned all thought of studying medicine forever; thereafter, when asked, I would say that I was going to study agronomy. I should add that I barely knew what agronomy was, but what I did know was that it was related to agriculture and – thanks to Robin – that Israel needed agronomists. However, by the time I enrolled in university in Jerusalem after my military service in 1962 I realized that I had absolutely no interest in agronomy, so decided instead to become a high school teacher of History and English. And, when I came to join the army, it is ironic that by sheer happenstance I eventually ended up as a combat medic, when there are so many other different branches of the military.

1960 was my final year of high school, and the year that I turned sixteen. (Being in the Southern hemisphere, the South African school year begins around January/February and ends around November.) That year, my brother Steve went to Israel on a one-year youth leadership course. This was every Habonim member's dream, and I was green with envy. He returned just as I was completing high school. I had been writing to him secretly urging him to persuade our parents to let me go on the youth leadership program.

When Steve returned, he and I sat down and had a solemn and serious discussion. We both vowed we would go and live in Israel and, with the impulsiveness and naiveté of youth, (Steve was nineteen and a half and I was three years younger), we decided to inform our parents right away, and to invite them to join us. And that is precisely what we did. We sat them down and announced that we had both decided to make Aliyah, and invited them to do the same. What is more, I informed them that I was not intending to study at a university in South Africa and then emigrate, as was the usual pattern with our friends in Habonim, but was planning on leaving just as soon as I had enough money to pay for my air ticket. They must have been immensely shocked and perhaps troubled, too, but to their eternal credit they did not show it. The more I think about this, the more remarkable I find their initial response and, even more so, their ultimate decision, for after giving it some days' thought they informed us that, in order to keep the family together, they would immigrate to Israel, too – all this without having any idea what awaited them there. Steve was the only one in the family who had ever visited the country and, as I have pointed out, my parents were not Zionists and were largely uninformed about Israel. What is more, they were far from wealthy, which was going to make immigration to the young and poor country of Israel very difficult; any thought of an exploratory trip was out of the question, as it would have eaten up too much of their meager savings. So, at the ages of 50 and 46 respectively, my father and mother agreed to make the move, burning their bridges in South Africa without ever having set foot in Israel.

The fact that my parents made Aliyah meant that Steve and I would have a family there, and would not be alone. In the event, my parents lived in Israel from 1961 – 1974, and we will always treasure the happy time we spent together in Jerusalem. And this was in spite of the fact that my parents worked much harder and life was much tougher in Jerusalem than it would have been had they stayed in Johannesburg.

Yet, despite their tough lives in still underdeveloped Israel, my mother told me, many years later, that the years they spent there were indeed the happiest of their lives.

We devised a plan. I would get a job in order to save up to pay for my air ticket, while Steve would study one more year at university in South Africa before joining us; my parents, for their part, would start planning their own emigration once I had left. I got a job as a clerk in an accounting firm owned by a distant cousin, and lasted there precisely one month – I absolutely hated it, despite having the goal of the ticket to Israel to encourage me. I then became a dispatch clerk and a salesman in a large furniture store in downtown Johannesburg. This work was more varied and interesting, and I actually quite enjoyed it, but that was partially due to the knowledge that it was temporary, and indeed after five months, by May of 1961, I'd saved up the money for the ticket. At the same time, I was in continual contact with the Aliyah officers at the South African Zionist Federation (The Jewish Agency), and when I was getting close to having sufficient money I asked them to arrange a place for me on a six-month 'ulpan' (a residential Hebrew course) on a kibbutz. There were several such courses offered on kibbutzes, and the plan was that you worked half a day in return for food and accommodation, and were taught and studied Hebrew for the other half day.

Towards the end of April I received a call from the Aliyah officer that a place had been reserved for me on the *ulpan* at Kibbutz Ma'ayan Zvi on the Mediterranean, north of Tel Aviv, and that the course would begin on June 1. I was ecstatic. My plan was to study for six months at the ulpan, and then go to university, after which I would do my army service, which at the time was two and a half years. I immediately gave notice at my job and planned to leave. Being only seventeen I had very few worldly possessions, and as far as I can remember all I bought was a pair of stout boots and a good sleeping bag. I always laugh when people aware of the strict currency controls in South Africa ask me whether I had trouble getting my money out – I had none whatsoever to bring out!

I booked an El Al Israel Airlines flight leaving Johannesburg on May 31, arriving in Tel Aviv the following day. At the time it was unsafe for

El Al planes to overfly certain countries in Africa which were extremely hostile to Israel and so, despite the flight, the crew, the food and even the magazines being El Al's, the actual plane in which we flew was a Sabena Airlines plane chartered by El Al. Its route dictated as much by security concerns as by the need to refuel, we flew Johannesburg – Leopoldville (today Kinshasa, in the Congo) – Athens – Tel Aviv. My departure date of May 31 was highly symbolic because on that exact day, in 1961, South Africa ceased to be a member of the Commonwealth and became a republic, thereby making it more of a pariah state than ever. I was overjoyed to be leaving.

On the flight with me were three fellow-South Africans enrolled in a special program for foreign volunteers in the Israeli army. They seemed nice enough, but little did I know that, within 24 hours, I would be a member of their group and headed, not for Kibbutz Ma'ayan Zvi and its *ulpan*, but rather, like them, for the Israeli army instead.

When the State of Israel was established in 1948, one of the first laws passed was the Law of Return, which entitled every Jew in the world to take out Israeli citizenship immediately on arrival in the country. Subsequently, under the same law, certain 'refuseniks' (from what was then the Soviet Union) were granted Israeli citizenship before ever being allowed to leave the Soviet Union. The alternative to taking out citizenship immediately for people like myself, who had left their country voluntarily, was to be a 'temporary resident' for three years, after which you were required to take out citizenship and serve in the army, or leave the country.

June 1 was a blazing hot summer's day. Here I was in Israel, having left my family and my life behind, although I did know that my family would soon be following me. It was early in the morning when we landed, and I was met by Amnon, the driver from the South African Zionist Federation offices. He took the South African volunteers and me to the Federation's offices on Hayarkon Street on the waterfront in Tel Aviv, where we were welcomed by Symie, an ex-South African who was employed by the 'Fed,' as the Zionist Federation was known. After some brief conversation, he directed me to the offices of the Jewish Agency, the body responsible for the different *ulpan* programs for immigrants. Once there, I was to inform them that I'd arrived and make arrangements for travel to Kibbutz Ma'ayan Zvi as soon as possible, since the *ulpan* had begun that day. I was given directions, and off I went, alone, 17 years of age and jet-lagged.

Bad news awaited me at the Jewish Agency offices. There I learned that they had no record of a place having been reserved for me at the Ma'ayan Zvi *ulpan*, that in any case it was now full and, worst of all, that there was no other course starting for several months. All this despite the South African Zionist Federation in Johannesburg having received a telegram from the Jewish Agency in Tel Aviv, informing them that a place was being held for me at Kibbutz Ma'Ayan Zvi in their *ulpan*, beginning June 1.

I was very young, very naïve and totally ignorant of how chaotic and bureaucratic things were in the Israel of those days. And I certainly did not know that, had I made enough of a fuss, a place would magically have been found for me. I had yet to learn how to assert myself in such situations – a skill that took me years to develop. I was, understandably, deeply worried. I had given up a job and emigrated on the basis of a guaranteed reservation at the kibbutz, and here I was, without a return ticket or the means of buying one, with all my plans in disarray and in the painful process of learning that in the Israel of the 1960s such plans and reservations did not necessarily guarantee anything. I listened to what they told me at the Jewish Agency, and decided to go back to the Fed to ask their advice.

And there Symie, the ex-South African, offered me a solution. There was this group of South Africans assembling in order to go into the army at the end of July to do their National Service as part of a special program, called 'Machal,' for 'foreign volunteers,' that is, people who volunteered to go into the army before they were conscripted. He suggested that I join them. What else could I do? I became a member of *Machal*, and thus encountered for a second time my fellow passengers of the night before.

The *Machal* program as it then existed was an outgrowth of the War of Independence of 1948, in which thousands of foreign volunteers – Jews from all over the world – rallied to the side of the fledgling State, and came to fight in the war. Many of these people brought invaluable military skills gained in the ranks of the Allied forces in World War Two – 'Machalniks,' for example, are credited with the creation of the Israeli Air Force.

From that glorious beginning *Machal* had developed into a program to entice young Jews to come to Israel (airfare and expenses paid) and serve in the army, in the hope that a number of them would then decide to settle permanently in the country. The program existed largely to attract what we called 'unaffiliated' youth – young people who were not members of Zionist youth movements, and therefore had little knowledge of, or contact with, Israel. So these boys (and a few girls) were seldom committed Zionists, and despite the intent of the program organizers, in truth very, very few of them had any intention of settling in Israel – they had signed up more for the fun of it than for anything else.

There were several powerful attractions to Symie's proposal that I join the *Machal* group preparing to enlist in the army with the next intake at the end of July. First, I would be serving with other South Africans. Granted, these men were not exactly the type of idealistic youth movement friends I had been mixing with, but the three I had met seemed nice enough. The second attraction was that, as a 'volunteer,' I would only be required to serve half the normal National Service that other Israelis served – fifteen months instead of the usual thirty. As a reluctant soldier I saw this as an opportunity to be done with military service in half the time. In addition to this, I would learn Hebrew while doing it. It would mean that I could begin university in the Fall of 1962 – albeit one year later than planned – but having completed my compulsory service. The final attraction was that I would be required to take on Israeli citizenship immediately, and the prospect of doing so, and thereby shedding the South African citizenship which had grown so distasteful to me, was most appealing. I was convinced.

It now remained for me to convince my parents to allow me to enlist, since being under 18 and by Israeli law still a minor, I needed parental consent. In those days, long distance calls from Israel to South Africa were unheard of – few Israelis had telephones, and anyway such calls were prohibitively expensive *if* one succeeded in getting through at all. I decided to send them a telegram explaining the situation, and awaited their response with trepidation. To my delight they agreed without any argument. I often wonder how my wife, Jenny, and I would have responded had one of our children at 17 first announced that they were emigrating, then invited us to follow, and finally followed this up with a request for permission to enlist as a volunteer. I am not at all sure that we would have been as accommodating as my parents were.

With my parents cabled permission in hand, on July 31 I began my service in a *Machal* group within the 'Nachal' ('Fighting Pioneering Youth') Regiment. There was an added and not insubstantial bonus to going into *Machal* immediately. Since this was a program to encourage young South Africans to settle in Israel, their airfare to Israel was paid, and they received an additional thirteen Israeli Lira per month salary from the South African Zionist Federation over and above the twelve we received from the army, plus two overseas air letters per week. Even I, who had joined the program in Israel, was eligible for this, so when I signed up I was, to my delight, reimbursed for my air fare. This was a fortune for me in those days, and was put to excellent use: it ultimately enabled me to buy a motor scooter shortly after finishing my service.

I made that fateful decision to go directly into the army on June 2, the day after I arrived in Israel. At 7.00 a.m. the following morning, with part of our South African *Machal* group I was taken to Jaffa for our medical examinations. Little did I know that these examinations would establish my health rating ('profil') for the rest of my army life, and that one's *profil* determined the type of unit (front-line combat, non-combat service, or other) in which one served. There were hundreds of people milling around, most carrying little glass yogurt bottles with different amounts of urine in them, while people in uniform would pop out of a room barking something unintelligible at us, to which we were supposed to respond – except that we were incapable of doing so, since none of us knew enough Hebrew to understand the orders. We followed gestured instructions, and were medically tested to a lesser or greater degree. The funniest part of the medical was having our photographs taken. We were sent down onto the street to be photographed by an old man with an even older camera of the type you see in silent movies, in which the photographer conceals himself under a cloth attached to the camera before taking the shot. We were seated, one by one, on a rickety old chair with a wooden pole nailed to the back of it, to which was attached a cloth "backdrop" of questionable cleanliness. After the photographer had taken the picture – good enough for any 'Wanted for Murder!' poster – we had to wait while he developed the picture in an old biscuit tin of chemicals. Ramshackle though the equipment may well have been with which this photograph was taken, the picture itself became part of a document of the utmost significance in my life, for it adorned such vital and essential pieces of identification as my army ID card and, subsequently, my reservist's ID card.

What we found when comparing notes at the end of that gruelling but at the same time amusing morning was that we had not all undergone the same medical tests. Some of us had been tested for hernia, but a urine sample had not been taken; some had had their hearing but not their vision tested, and on and on. I, for one, never had my eyes tested, and so despite the fact that I already wore relatively strong glasses, I served throughout my military career with a health rating of '97,' the highest you can get – an impossibility if you wear glasses. Well, nothing is impossible when you are as ignorant as we were.

That very same day I also took out Israeli citizenship. As momentous an event in my life as this was, in many ways it was something of an anticlimax. All that happened was that I was required to sign some papers – no pomp, no ceremony, no anthem. Paradoxically, receiving Canadian citizenship some twenty years later was a much more moving moment because of the ceremony we attended. Nor was my ceasing to have valid South African citizenship at that moment any more stirring, because there was no act of renunciation or dramatic surrendering of my passport: I simply was no longer legally eligible to hold one. But still, that was quite a lot to have happen in one day to a jet-lagged seventeen-year old who did not speak the language.

The three men who were on the plane with me from South Africa were by no means the vanguard of the new *Machal* group, as several others had already arrived and had been placed on Kibbutz Hasolelim near Nazareth. This was where our group was mustered over the months of June and July before actually being inducted on July 31. On the kibbutz we worked and learned some Hebrew, an identical set-up, in fact, to a kibbutz *ulpan*, with half the day for work and the other half for Hebrew lessons. It was bakingly hot, and we did back-breaking work, mainly harvesting the sugar beet, which had us working doubled over either to cut the greenery off the tops one day, or to throw the uprooted beets onto a slowly moving truck another day. This was my first encounter with serious physical labor, and it took some getting used to. Moreover, I decided on one of my first days to take off my shirt to get cooler, got terribly badly sunburned, and was in agony. Sunscreen was unheard of in those days and, in any case, even if it did exist, as it very probably did, real men didn't use it.

While we were on Hasolelim, we were taken on a week's visit to Jerusalem to be shown all the major sights. We were taken to the Knesset – the Israeli parliament – which at that time met in a building on King George Street at the top of Ben Yehuda Street. We sat in the visitors' area for a short while observing the proceedings, none of which we could understand. It did, however give me a certain thrill to know that I, a citizen, was observing the members of parliament of the Jewish state, my state, in session.

Two visits stand out most of all for me. One was to the Mandelbaum Gate, which was the only official crossing point in divided Jerusalem, between Israeli West Jerusalem and Jordanian East Jerusalem, where the Old City and the Western Wall were. (Israel and Jordan at that point were still in a state of war, and no crossing was allowed in either direction by either Israelis or Jordanians – each half of the city was totally out of bounds to the other. The only people who were allowed to cross were diplomats, U.N. officials and Christian pilgrims. We were most intrigued by the fact that we were standing inches from Jordan and could see Jordanian police and officials just a few feet away. I never thought at that moment I would one day be fighting a war against them.) However, almost immediately after East Jerusalem and the Old City were liberated by *Tzahal* during the Six Day War and Jerusalem was reunited, all vestiges of the crossing point were obliterated, and for a long time it has been difficult to find the exact spot where the gate had stood. Today when I visit Israel, every time I am in that area, I still think back to the days when the city was divided, and I think, too, of all that followed in the Six Day War. Today, a gas station called 'Mandelbaum' stands just there, and a small monument, located on a traffic island in the middle of a major highway joining the Old City and Mount Scopus with the northern suburbs of Jerusalem, marks the exact point where the border used to be.

The second visit was to the end of Jaffa Road, where we peered through the hole in the wall marking the border into Jordanian East Jerusalem, and to Kibbutz Ramat Rachel which, lying to the south of Jerusalem, was the closest point to Bethlehem. Today, Kibbutz Ramat Rachel has been swallowed up by urban sprawl, and much of its agricultural land has been sold to Jerusalem's urban developers. As I stood there on that day 41 years ago, I could not have imagined that I would get married in Jerusalem, make my home in Jerusalem, fight in Jerusalem and in 2001 attend the wedding of my daughter Noa in a beautiful reception hall right there at Kibbutz Ramat Rachel.

I did not give much thought to the fact that Jerusalem was a divided city; after all, this was the only reality that I knew. And even when later I lived there we rarely reflected on this, except when there were exchanges of fire across the urban line, or when we visited lookout points from which we could view the 'other side' of the city, or when we heard stories of earlier times. Our feeling about the fact that Jerusalem was divided was, therefore, very different from that of veteran Israelis who had known Jerusalem as a united city, and had perhaps lived in the Old City, or studied at the Hebrew University on Mount Scopus, and prayed at the Western Wall.

The other memorable part of our week in Jerusalem was a forty-five minute visit to the Eichmann Trial being held at the converted Beit Ha'am Theater on Bezalel Street. The theater had been converted into a court specially for the trial. The proceedings were in Hebrew, with Eichmann and others responding in German, so we were loaned devices to enable us to follow the proceedings through a simultaneous translation into English. This was not a dramatic part of the trial – the Chief Prosecutor, Gideon Hausner, was cross-examining Eichmann about technical matters relating to train schedules, but still, having been there, in the same room with that man, was simply unforgettable.

There stood Eichmann, the personification of evil, looking like any middle-aged, balding individual. He was calm and answered Hausner's questions in a totally dispassionate, almost self-satisfied manner. So much so that sitting there observing this, it was not hard to forget the ghoulishness of the crime for which this man was being tried. No doubt it was entirely different when a survivor like Ka-Tzetnik 135633, (the *nom de plume* of a concentration camp survivor-author meaning "Prisoner number 135633"), was giving his evidence.

And, on July 31, I duly began my army service. I was young, idealistic and starry-eyed, and to realize that I was serving in the army of the thirteen-year old State of Israel – the country I had decided to make my home – sent thrills down my spine. When I looked at myself in the uniform of the Defense Army of Israel, I swelled with pride. In fact, one of the first things I did when I got leave in basic training was to go to a professional studio and have my picture taken in uniform.

Several years before emigrating from South Africa, I had vowed that I would never serve in the South African Army because it was used as a reserve force to the police in suppressing and oppressing the blacks, and I was not willing to be a part of that endeavor. Serving in the Israeli Army was a very different proposition. This was an honorable and noble thing to do, much as I disliked all things military. I knew that it was not chance that led to its name being 'The Defense Army of Israel,' and that *Tzahal* existed to defend the State of Israel whose existence has consistently been challenged by its neighbors ever since Independence in 1948.

I was never a good athlete, being always a bit on the heavy side, and was somewhat nervous about basic training and the physical demands that would be made of me. Mind you, I wasn't that bad, either – many were worse. I followed orders, managed the physical demands more or less successfully, and learned the basic things that a simple soldier needs to learn. Most important, I learned what I believe are the two most important aspects to being a soldier: to obey orders without questioning, and to guard my rifle "as if it were my wife."

We were trained in infantry combat, and then stationed on the border. This was the basic plan of the *Nachal* Regiment in which we served, by which Zionist youth movement graduates like me, both Israelis and immigrants, would serve part of their time on a border kibbutz, and ultimately make the kibbutz their home. Though enchanted by life on a kibbutz, and while there even talking of making my home on one, my life ultimately followed different twists and turns and I never did return to kibbutz life after being discharged.

During the two months we spent on Kibbutz Hasolelim we got to know each other, and friendships formed. We worked hard in the sugar beet fields, were taken on several trips around the country, and learned some Hebrew. An enjoyable interlude, and one which left us looking forward to joining up and serving together in the army at the end of July.

The night before we were inducted we were all transferred to Tel Aviv, ready to be taken the following morning to the Induction Center. A group of us decided to do something we thought very daring. First we went to one of Tel Aviv's most famous haunts, the Mugrabi Cinema, to see *David and Batsheva*; we then ate a hamburger and finally, in our last civilian act of defiance, strolled down to the beach in front of the Dan Hotel and went skinny-dipping. It was pitch dark, and there was no one else around, for the Tel Aviv beach in those days was a pretty unsavory place – literally so, for as far as I could ascertain raw sewage flowed directly into the sea nearby. Nothing, moreover, had at that stage been done to beautify the beachfront in any way. Since then, however, the beach has been completely cleaned up, and a handsome boardwalk stretches for miles along the Mediterranean, virtually all the way from downtown Tel Aviv to Jaffa. Although there was not a soul around, we still felt we had done something exceptionally daring.

I entered the army in a group of some 40 young people, 37 men and 3 women. (The women went through a much easier and shorter basic training, and served separately from the men, only rejoining us when we went to the kibbutz after basic training. In those days women did not serve in combat units at all, performing such duties as clerks, nurses and radio operators.) Thirty-nine of us were ex-South Africans, and the single most noticeable feature of our group was our almost total lack of any knowledge of Hebrew. This may sound like a major disadvantage. In fact we quickly realized that we could turn it to our advantage and, on that very first day en route in a military transport from the Induction Center to our base, we made a pact that even when we did understand, we would make as if we did not. This, as I said, not only worked to our advantage, but bonded us together, so that we came through many difficult and stressful situations rolling with laughter, due to our conspiracy of linguistic ignorance.

At the Induction Center we were issued our uniforms, kitbags, mess tins, boots, and other necessities of army life, and were told to change into uniform. We weren't even given real underwear, but instead were issued with hilarious garments reminiscent of apparel our grandfathers might have worn: coarse cotton, boxer-style, and held up not with anything as modern and newfangled as elastic, but with a drawstring. This underwear had been confiscated from Egyptian military stores in the Sinai Desert during the Sinai Campaign of 1956. I don't think any of us ever wore it. The boots we were issued were also of poor quality, made from coarse leather, and they, like the underwear, had been "liberated" in the Sinai Campaign. With soles made from what looked like old car tires, and nailed into place, these monstrosities did not, as my friends were soon to learn, last long. Mine, and my friend Jackie's, were different – we had the largest feet of our group, and with our foot size the boots were not rubber-soled but hobnailed, that is, studded with projections like nail-heads. Initially, we thought nothing of this strange difference in army issue footwear ...

We were then told to line up in single file and to roll up our sleeves. As we approached the head of the line, we realized that there were two medics, one to our left, one to our right, and as we passed them, they each gave us a shot in the arm simultaneously – one, I know, was anti-tetanus, but I never did find out what the other was. But we were now ready to set off for our basic training camp. Remember, it was just two months since I had arrived in Israel, so when we were told where the base was it meant nothing to me, nor indeed to most of us. We, together with all our equipment, were loaded into an open military truck (no seats, so we sat on our kitbags) and we set off for basic training, not having a clue what awaited us.

After traveling for some time, the truck stopped outside the gates of a large army base. A plump, sweaty sergeant, who closely resembled a bulldog, was waiting, hands on hips, and he began barking orders at us in Hebrew. I was soon to learn that hands on hips was the most common stance of anyone with any rank in *Tzahal*, making me think I had landed in a Hollywood war movie. We understood enough to grasp that he was ordering us to get off the truck with all our equipment and to line up in threes. It was not that easy to get down from the truck with everything we had to carry, and it took us time. And then we realized by the way Bulldog was looking at his watch that it had taken us too long. He then gave us three minutes to load everything *back* onto the truck and then to offload it again and to line up. This caused total pandemonium as we all scrambled to get on and then off the truck at once and, needless to say, Bulldog was far from satisfied, and we had to do it again. I have no idea how many times we jumped on and off that truck, but it seemed to be dozens, although I doubt it was more than three or four.

When Bulldog was finally satisfied, he had us do a right turn and then ordered us to run in formation. And that was how we entered the base. It was not that easy to run with all our equipment and parcels, but run we did. The roads in the camp were paved, and when we reached our destination he barked, "Halt!" Well, all the small-footed, rubber-shod people duly halted, while Jackie and I, with our hobnails, went flying into the rest of the group. And that was what happened to the two of us almost every time we were brought to a sudden halt on a paved road until, to our relief, the hobnails fell off our boots and they became ordinary leather soles.

But there were also compensations for being so large: Jackie and I were both over 1.80 metres tall, and we heard a rumor that if you were that height, you were entitled to double rations. This proved to be absolutely true – it was a carry-over from the *Tzena*, the period of austerity in the first years of the State, when there was not enough food available, and there was food rationing for everyone. By 1961, when we went into the army, there was ample food always, but not very generous helpings of meat or fruit, for example. Moreover, the food was predictably boring – breakfast, for example, was *invariably* very hard boiled eggs, spring onions, olives, bread and tea/coffee – beverages usually indistinguishable in taste. So Jackie and I went off to see the medical officer, as we were entitled to do, and he measured us and issued each of us with a piece of paper instructing mess staff to issue us with double rations. What a treat! It made the hobnails seem well worthwhile.

Before we had even been inducted we had heard of the legendary 'Terror' of our base camp – the Sergeant Major! It is astounding that somehow the warning had reached us, even on the kibbutz, to beware of the Sergeant Major. Well, no sooner had we screeched to a halt than the Terror came sauntering up, swagger stick under his arm, to 'greet' and terrorize us. He began pacing up and down in front of our group and then asked, "Who speaks Hebrew?"

Not a response – the conspiracy was holding. After repeating the question several times with different speeds and ever ampler gestures, he then asked, in Yiddish, "Who speaks Yiddish?"

In the fiercely proud thirteen-year-old State of Israel, this nation of 'new Jews' who fought back and never turned the other cheek or lowered their gaze, the use of Yiddish was frowned on. None of the younger Israelis used it at all because of its association with the days of anti-Semitism in Europe, a past we hoped was behind us forever, with its dreadful associations with the hideously anti-Semitic countries of Eastern Europe, where Jews had been so horribly oppressed. (Of course it remained the lingua franca of many elderly European Jews, and of ultra Orthodox Jews who regarded Hebrew as the sacred language of prayer.) So for this bully, a Sergeant Major in the Israeli Army, to have to resort to Yiddish certainly took the wind out of his sails. Harry, the clown of the group, raised his hand and explained that he spoke "a bissel" (a bit) and that his "Bobba in Drom Africa" (his Granny in South Africa) had taught him. We just exploded with laughter, much to the anger of Terror, who screamed at us to be quiet, and then proceeded to give us our 'welcoming' talk, or should I say to issue a stream of orders and threats, in Yiddish, translated very poorly by Harry as we all chortled. I should confess at this point that I already knew a little Hebrew – enough to understand commands like "Run!"

"Sit!" and "Be on the parade ground in three minutes!" and the like, but a pact is a pact, and I never let on. I think we were the only group of new inductees who were not cowed by Terror on that first day. Moreover, we had learned that by causing officers to explain things to us in English, which was not always so easy for them, we were able to cast them in an inferior and therefore less threatening role for us. We exploited this to the full and also had a lot of fun with it.

For example, one day we all felt we had had just about enough of officers standing on the parade ground saying things like, "On the word "up," you have two minutes to bring your beds onto the parade ground." (This was said in Hebrew, and for some reason it was always, "On the word "up" – or maybe it was "hup"…) Well, on this particular day we just did not want to be performing circus lions, because that is what the "On the word "up"" order sounded like to us. So, when we were told, "On the word "up," you have two minutes to bring your beds onto the parade ground," we all raised our hands just as circus lions or performing dogs would do with their front paws, and let out a roar. Our officer had the grace to burst out laughing.

Our ignorance and naiveté was so great that now I can only marvel at its very profundity. For example, at the end of our first week in the army, we were given leave for the weekend to take our civilian gear home. We were highly excited. The first week had been grueling, with officers waking us sometimes every hour on the hour throughout the night, and then putting us through long and strenuous days in the blazing heat. After morning inspection and parade, we were given our passes and told we could go. Most of us were heading to Tel Aviv. We went out to the main road, *but had no idea where we were and in which direction we should be heading, let alone how far we were from Tel Aviv.* I think it is a tribute to our ingenuity that we eventually found our way there and then back again to the base on the Sunday morning.

Most of what I remember about basic training relates to my virtually non-existent Hebrew, the physical demands made on us, and things like that. But there was one crowning moment, which stands out above all the others – the moment we were given our rifles.

New recruits in *Tzahal* are always given their first rifles at some sort of ceremony. We received ours at a special torchlight parade a couple of weeks into basic training. At the same moment as being handed the rifle, we were each given a Bible with *Tzahal's* crest on it. An oath of allegiance was read out on our behalf and then, as we received the rifle and Bible, we were required to say in Hebrew, "I swear." In Habonim, we had learned all about the birth of the State of Israel, and how the Jews had had to struggle against much larger and better equipped forces, and how hard it had been for them to procure and then keep arms to which they weren't legally entitled during the British Mandate government in pre-independence years. Rifles are precious in any army, and growing to appreciate their importance is an essential feature of good soldiery, but this special ceremony made the receiving of a rifle, legally and from *Tzahal*, the army of the Jewish state, all the more important and symbolic. All my Zionist education and dreams and love of Israel came flooding into my head that night, and I was moved to tears.

Less than two weeks after basic training began, my parents left South Africa for their new lives in Israel, and I was granted special leave to go and meet them at the airport and spend a few days with them. I was told to report to a certain office on the base to get my pass. Now the army's idea of order, indeed maybe even of beauty, is raked sand, as found in front of an officer's quarters – sand raked into straight lines and enclosed for even better effect within a frame of whitewashed stones – a sort of military alternative to a flower bed. Although my officers knew I was in a rush to leave in order to make it to the airport to meet my parents, I was held back through morning parade and inspection. As you can imagine, when I was finally told to go and collect my pass I was in a frantic rush, ran straight across one of those raked squares – and straight into the arms of an officer. Although I knew exactly what I'd done wrong, it was only my professed total incomprehension of my misdeed that saved me from punishment.

By the time I was finally issued my pass, had raced to the camp gate and out on to the road to hitchhike to the airport, it was too late and I knew that I would miss my parents' arrival. I was as upset about this as I was sure they would be. However we'd had the foresight to discuss contingency plans in case I was not granted leave, so instead of going to the airport I hitchhiked to the residential *ulpan*, Ulpan Ben Yehuda in Netanya, where I knew they were being sent and which was not too far away. Ulpan Ben Yehuda was brand new and this was the first course to be held there. The houses had just been built, and there was no grass anywhere – the houses' foundations rested on sea sand.

I arrived minutes after my parents. They had been met by the faithful Amnon from the South African Zionist Federation, the same driver who had met me on my arrival, and he had brought them directly to the *ulpan*.

This was a heartfelt but, in some respects, a surreal reunion – there we were in the blazing Israeli sun, in a tiny little house built literally on the very sand dunes of the Mediterranean (but sadly without any ocean view) in a strange land of whose language my parents were completely ignorant, all of us having burned our bridges by coming to Israel, and me, the younger son, in army uniform. As I think back to that day 40 years ago, I consider my parents truly heroic. They had left a lovely suburban house in Johannesburg, with full time domestic help in both home and garden, the latter immaculately tended, and what they came to was a place without a blade of grass, let alone a flower, indeed without even the shelter of an inch of shade. And they were doing it all for the sake of keeping our family together.

Immediately my parents had made the decision to leave for Israel they had put their home in Johannesburg on the market. Unfortunately, as luck would have it, there was a major slump in the property market just then, and by the time they left it had still not been sold. My uncle eventually found them a tenant for just over a year, after which he managed to sell it for them, but for substantially less than they had paid for it ten years previously.

As a result of being unable to sell their home, my parents arrived with pitifully little capital, and my father was desperately anxious about how they would manage. My mother, on the other hand, was more philosophical, or perhaps she just managed to hide her anxiety better. Either way, they decided to be frugal with what they spent until they had jobs and were earning again. This meant a decision, for example, for these two heavy smokers to smoke only 'Silon' cigarettes, the very cheapest and, I am told, really foul-tasting. The residential *ulpan* was heavily subsidized by the Jewish Agency, so that the cost of their housing, food and tuition was most reasonable, and they did not have many other expenses during those first six months.

The biggest impact that this worry about the future had on them was that my father was unable to concentrate on his Hebrew studies – he was much too worried about finding a job – and as a result, he did not make as much progress as he might have. I have subsequently studied this phenomenon both from a theoretical and an empirical standpoint in my professional life, and have seen many immigrants do precisely what he did. My father had to take off numerous days from class in order to go for job interviews, and when he was in class job anxiety sapped his energy, diverting his attention from his language learning.

Life for them at the *ulpan* was not easy – the house was minute, and there were not even refrigerators – only ice-boxes, and every day a man with a donkey and cart came around selling blocks of ice. True, they had their meals in a communal dining room, but still, to have gone back after years of electric refrigeration to the humble ice-box was quite a shock.

However my parents were remarkable – they simply were not complainers. I am reminded of an incident that occurred on that first day at their *ulpan*. My mother was a woman obsessed with cleanliness – both personal cleanliness and the cleanliness of her home. When they reached the *ulpan* in Netanya they had been on the go for over twenty four hours, and my mother immediately announced that she was going to have a bath. She turned on the water in the tub, and it made quite a noise as it came gushing out. My father at this moment was in the little living room, and called to my mother over the noise of the water: "Well, Hilary, what is your first impression of Israel?"

Over the noise of the water, my mother replied, "I'm appalled!"

The rushing of the water made it difficult for my father to hear her exact words, and he responded triumphantly, "I *knew* you'd like it!"

This event occurred in 1961. My father died in 1975 and it was only in the early 1980s, some twenty years later, that my mother chose to tell us this story, confessing that she'd never told anyone until then, least of all my father.

Although the transition for my parents from affluent suburban Johannesburg to life in the *ulpan* was difficult, they felt that they had taken the first essential step towards re-establishing our home in Israel, and that was the most important thing for them. What also made it all much easier was the wonderful group of immigrants who studied at the *ulpan* with them. Many of these people were also from South Africa, and there was a great deal of socializing, bonding, and of people helping each other and functioning as surrogate relatives to replace those who had been left behind.

My parents' persistence in seeking work paid off, however, and by the time the *ulpan* finished they both had jobs in Jerusalem. My father, who had been the comptroller of a large firm in Johannesburg, was hired to work in the accounts department of Friedman's, manufacturers of kerosene stoves, refrigerators, and more. My mother was hired as an English secretary in the Israel Government Tourist Corporation – what was to become the Ministry of Tourism. My dad's job was well below the level to which he was accustomed, and my mother found herself back in secretarial work, something she had been very happy to give up many years earlier in order to work as a nursery school teacher. But they were thrilled, as this was the next step of their master plan

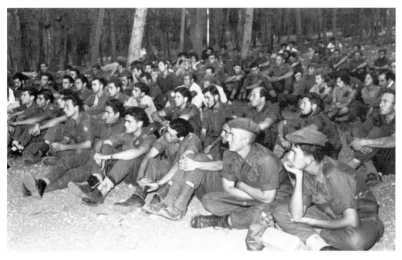

At a picnic for South African immigrants to Israel, Ben Shemen Forest, 1961. I am sitting in the front row right, looking pensive.

duly achieved. The moment they received their first pay checks, they upgraded the cigarettes they smoked – a very telling touch.

After my couple of days' leave I returned to basic training, and only saw my parents about every four weeks. At the camp we South Africans slowly settled into a routine, gradually becoming accustomed to the physical demands made on new recruits and the way in which they are treated. Nevertheless, throughout the three and a half months of basic training, we continued to play our 'I don't understand' card most effectively.

All of us South Africans used to give our letters to mail in town to anyone going on leave so that they would reach their destinations more quickly by evading the military censors. One day a fellow South African, a friend of mine named Ivan, was caught depositing a whole mass of our letters in a civilian mail box in Tel Aviv, precisely in order to achieve these two desirable goals of speed and confidentialty. The regulations, which we knew full well, required that all mail be handed in at the base and screened by the military censors, but then it took a week or longer to reach its destination. It was not that any of us wanted to send any secret information – frankly, we had none to divulge anyway – it was just the matter of speed. Ivan had committed a serious breach of military security, punishable by a term in military prison, an open and shut case as he was apprehended, in uniform, by a military policeman precisely at the very moment that he was dropping the letters into the mail box. He was promptly arrested and taken to a military lock-up. Remembering the rules of the game, all Ivan kept saying in Hebrew was, "Ani Ivrit katan. Ani lo mevin." ("I am just a small Hebrew. I don't understand." Ivan was anything but small, by the way.) He was let off with a stern warning.

There were many very funny aspects to doing basic training in this fog of linguistic incomprehension. For example, when they began teaching us about the rifle, the first thing we had to do was to memorize the name for each of the parts. This is not that difficult a task in one's first language, but to us it was very difficult, and we were often punished for confusing the names of parts. I am convinced that our officers thought that we were dim-witted because it took us so long to learn the parts. And that made us fall victim to the army's educational philosophy of "What you don't learn through the head, you will learn through the feet." Or, to paraphrase: "If you don't know what we have taught you, then we will give you physical punishments like push-ups." We ultimately did learn the names of the parts and to this day I can flawlessly recite the names of the parts of a rifle in Hebrew, but not in English. Mind you, whenever I recall those lessons on the names of the parts of the rifle, I am reminded of the British poet Henry Reed's famous poem, *Naming of Parts*, which eloquently addresses this very topic. The first verse begins:

Today we have naming of parts. Yesterday
We had daily cleaning. And tomorrow,
We shall have what to do after firing. But today,
Today we have naming of parts.

The poem then goes on to actually name the different parts of the rifle, and is very clever indeed. It makes me think that Henry Reed and I must have pondered the same whimsical question: Why is it so important for a field soldier to be able to name the parts of his rifle?

Then there were the days on which we had lectures on military topics. In true military fashion, it meant a whole day of lectures, *and we just could not understand what they were saying*. This resulted, at times, in several of us falling asleep during these endless lectures; each time that we did, we were taken out and made to run around the parade ground a few times with our rifles above our heads. As if this would help us understand! We didn't really mind because we were fit, and the break from the tedium of the incomprehensible lectures was even welcome.

Even funnier was the first time we were taken for shooting practice. To reduce the possibility of accidents, in the Israeli army soldiers on live firing exercises are required to repeat the commands they are given about when to open fire, with how many rounds, at which target, and so on. But *we didn't understand* what we were required to repeat. So at first we kept quiet, only to be punished because we had been explicitly told we must repeat the orders. As a result what developed sounded something like this, which I'll relate in English, although of course it was in Hebrew:

Officer: "Three rounds... "
The South Africans: "eee ounds"
Officer: "At the targets in front of you ..."
The South Africans: "het de tots ifroovyu…"
Officer: "Fire!"
The South Africans: "Fire!"

It evoked memories of our school choir, and how some of the boys would mumble something vaguely resembling the words when they could not remember them.

Despite many humorous incidents in basic training the training itself was anything but light hearted and amusing, being singularly tough both physically and mentally. The guiding philosophy, common to all armies the world over, was to break down any inclination to refuse, ignore or resist orders, and then to build you up as a fighting man who would never question an order. This was done by being very hard on us, particularly at the beginning, and to come down savagely on anyone who even looked as if they might be inclined to disobey an order. This meant strict discipline and tough physical demands. Not everyone who is conscripted is able to take the physical and mental pressure, and suicides are not unheard of in basic training.

On one occasion in my unit we were on a very fast route march, essentially a forced march carrying full packs. One of the things that I found rather sadistic and difficult to justify was that we were never told in advance how long the march or the run – held outside the base and along the side of the road – would be, and on numerous occasions would be marched or run to the gates of the camp. Then, just when we thought we were turning into the camp and the strain was over, they would tell us to continue on straight ahead. This was especially hard on those who were having trouble. On that particular day it was officially a march, not a run, although the officer who led us was walking so fast that every one of us had to run all the way to keep up with him.

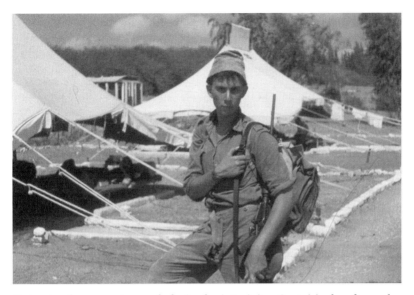

Returning from a route march during basic training. Surprisingly, after such a gruelling march, I look quite spry.

I, for one, was really struggling and praying it would soon be over. All of a sudden, I saw a man just in front of me move out of formation towards the center of the road, and try and throw himself under a passing truck. Luckily, one of our sergeants saw what he was doing and managed to push him out of the way of the truck, and he was unhurt.

Not only was discipline strict, but there also existed what I would translate literally as 'water discipline' or, more precisely, water rationing. At the time of the War of Independence in 1948, not only was Jerusalem under siege and water strictly rationed, but *Tzahal* often found it difficult and dangerous to get water to the different units in the field. As a result, there developed the philosophy that soldiers must learn to manage with very little water – usually with the litre or so of water that they carried in their personal canteens. I was to feel the full impact of the 'water discipline' on one of our route marches.

We were taken on an extremely tough two-day route march in the Galilee, and the packs with which we were burdened were the heaviest we had been required to carry up to this point. I would estimate that they weighed forty to fifty pounds. We would march for about 50 minutes and then rest for about ten. We were explicitly told that we were not allowed to drink any water until the order had been given. And even then, the order was something like – "Take one gulp only." It was mid-summer, blazing hot, with little shade anywhere.

During the first morning I was parched, and although we were on break the order to drink had not been given. I decided to have some water when the officers were not looking – or so I thought. One of my officers saw me, and for punishment he poured out the remainder of the water in my canteen, leaving me with no water for several hours. The going was tough, the packs were like lead, and it was stiflingly hot – well above thirty degrees Celsius. A couple of hours after this incident, I fainted. The officers splashed water in my face, picked me up and made me carry on. About an hour later I fainted again, and the same procedure was followed. I realize now that I was dehydrated and suffering from sunstroke. I made it through the day, and the following morning I set off with everyone else for day two of this awful march. About an hour into the morning, I fainted yet again, and this time the officers decided that I must be ill. They radioed for a jeep to come and get me and, much to my relief, I was taken back to the base. As far as I can recall, I was not seen by a doctor, but the fact that I could drink as much as I wanted, rest, and be in the shade, made all the difference.

The rest of the soldiers returned to the base late that afternoon. It was a Thursday, and we were due to go on leave the following morning for the weekend. On the Friday morning we got up, and prepared for daily inspection prior to being given our passes. On the parade ground my name was called out and I was told to report to a particular officer immediately. He informed me that my punishment for not completing the march was that my leave had been cancelled. I was devastated, but there was nothing I could do about it. I could not even call to let my parents know, so I sent a message to them with another soldier who was going to Netanya.

I do not believe that an incident like that would occur today, and if it did there would be recourse to the army ombudsman. In any case, the water policy, as I will describe later, was subsequently totally reversed.

I am happy to say that one of the features of *Tzahal* which sets it apart from what seems to be the case in, say, the U.S. Army – or at least the way that army is depicted in movies and books – is the absence of bullying. Yes, we were shouted at, but there was none of the screaming in your face that is present in every depiction of the U.S. Army, nor any individual humiliations; I never saw a recruit reduced to tears or cowering before an officer in fear.

Of course there were punishments, and many of them. But they tended to be meted out to the whole platoon, and usually took such forms as additional running around the parade ground or as extensions to the evening run, or being required to rush back and forth carrying our beds out to the parade ground in a fixed amount of time. Individual punishments were generally imposed by a senior officer at a formal hearing, after a proper charge had been laid, and were suitably documented.

In my own platoon, there was one incident that I recall vividly, and that was on Yom Kippur – one of the holiest days in the Jewish calendar. That is the day on which Jews fast from sunset to the following sunset, spending the day in the synagogue praying and asking for forgiveness for sins committed over the past year. The idea is that this is the final 'day of reckoning,' after which God decides who shall live and who shall die, and the accounts are closed. We did not have any training that day, and we were allowed to spend it praying and fasting or just resting in our tents. Well, one of our corporals, out of sheer spite, ordered us onto the parade ground in the middle of the afternoon. Today, if such a thing occurred, the noncommissioned officer would himself be put on a charge.

Another feature of life in *Tzahal* which I found interesting was the way in which individuals related to each other. I had attended an all-boys' high school, and it was not uncommon for a fist fight to develop out of an argument. Based on this experience and my literature-based knowledge of armies, I expected there to be a fair amount of fighting in the ranks. I was completely wrong. Israelis are intensely aggressive in their personal relations, if one can make national generalizations, but in spite of the noise that they make and the way they are liable to insult each other verbally, they seldom resort to physical violence. I witnessed several incidents in which two soldiers would have an argument, which quickly escalated into a shouting match and an exchange of insults. However, just at the point where I expected them to begin fighting, I would hear, "Hold me! I'm going to hit him!" and that was as far as the fighting went. It was often a very funny scene because the person shouting "Hold me" was often *looking* for someone to restrain them.

Physical conditions were tough. We slept in large tents, ten to a tent, and there was no electric lighting. The tents had concrete floors, which had to be swept and washed meticulously for daily inspection, but there were no containers for bringing water to the tent. It was up to us to work something out. In my tent, we managed to get hold of a large biscuit tin and we used that, but it was not that convenient as it had no handle. The result was that we ended up awkwardly carrying this tin with jagged edges backwards and forwards from the ablution block, and a fair amount of the water tended to be spilled out by the time we reached our tent.

While we had plenty of food, it was boring and unappealing. Lunch and supper were as tedious and uninviting as breakfast, or perhaps even more so. There was usually a sort of stewed meat, with potatoes. The amount of meat was minuscule, as meat in those days in Israel was prohibitively expensive, and of wretched quality to boot. All the food was strictly kosher, and there was a man stationed in every kitchen checking that the dietary laws were being adhered to.

Going to meals, like everything else, was done when the order was given. We were lined up in threes by platoon before every meal, and marched to our company's dining room. A corporal supervised our orderly entry into the British-built Nissen hut, with its typical semi-circular roof, and similarly our behavior in the line as we waited to be served. The men who served us always seemed to resent what they were doing, delighting in grumpily plopping the food into our mess tins, mixing it all up, and making it even less appealing than it could have been. Only the new recruits ate in these huts – all other ranks ate in a different mess, and I once noticed that they were even given plastic plates. That would indeed have been a luxury for us.

Kitchen duty was another unwelcome feature of basic training. As far as I can remember, I only had to do it twice, and disliked it both times. When I was told that I would be spending the whole of the following day working in the kitchen, I was quite pleased as I saw this as a day off hard physical training. However, when I arrived at the kitchen,

I quickly realized that I would prefer to be running, climbing, shooting, or whatever. The kitchen staff were regular army, and were a group of exceptionally unpleasant, frustrated men. Basically, they had one of the worst jobs in the whole of *Tzahal*, suffered on-going abuse from virtually all the men they cooked for, were not given any respect by their superiors, and were wretchedly paid.

When we arrived, the first thing that happened was that we had to hand in our rifles, which were then locked in a closet. I found this strange, but it was explained to me that this was to stop recruits from running away from kitchen duty. The logic was that if you were caught without your rifle you would be severely punished, so as long as our rifles were in the hands of the cooks our presence in the kitchen, however unwilling, was guaranteed. This was a poor start for any working relationship, and then to be shouted at all day by these men while, for example, we peeled mountains of cooked eggplant, virtually up to our elbows in it, was not my idea of a fun time.

We were given one set of fatigues per week – this was a pair of pants and a shirt, which had been some soldier's dress uniform when he was doing his national service – and we wore these, day and night, for a full week before being allowed to change them. When that day came, our fatigues were so filthy that they could have walked to the laundry room by themselves. It was mid-summer, we all sweated profusely, and what is more, we were only given time to shower about every 10 days. I found myself using substantial amounts of deodorant. However, in young Israel, real pioneers did not use deodorant – it was thought to be the clearest possible indication of a distinct lack of manliness. Nevertheless, in due course the deodorant I had brought from South Africa ran out. With no leave in the offing I asked another soldier, who had the enviable ability of always being able to wangle spots of leave usually on compassionate grounds, to buy me some next time he left camp. He brought me back a little stick of locally made deodorant, which had rather a pleasant smell. Delighted, I applied it with gusto, only to find that it stung terribly and frothed into a lather under my arms.

The *Machal* unit in which I served can only be described as a motley crew. Few were products of either a Zionist youth movement or a Zionist education, which meant that they weren't in either Israel or the army out of conviction or idealism. In fact, several of them were young men who had had problems of one sort or another in South Africa and did not know where their lives were going, and whose parents had thought that this army experience would straighten them out. Several, for example, had dropped out of or had never entered university, a somewhat unusual state of affairs for a Jew in South Africa at that time. I believe only a handful remained in Israel after demobilization, and from that point of view the program was, to my mind, something of a failure. But although I fell into it because of a chapter of accidents, it served my purposes well. I was quite a few years younger than most of the South Africans with whom I served, and had had a very different experience in my teen years thanks to Habonim. However, I got on well with most of them.

As much as I would describe some of the men in our platoon as real characters, the truth is we were basically a group of pretty well brought up South African kids, and we seldom got into serious trouble. There were, however, a few instances in which I myself was put on a charge for violating military regulations. Two of these occurred after I had completed basic training and was stationed on a kibbutz, but the first occurred during basic training:

One night, after we had completed our training for the night and had been told we could go to bed, a number of us were dying for something sweet to eat, such as a candy or a chocolate bar. We knew that there was a civilian kiosk across the main road outside the fence surrounding the camp. It was dark, so we decided to climb over the fence and go and buy something. Unfortunately, just as we were straddling the fence with one foot on either side, we were caught by one of our corporals who was passing by. Talk about smoking guns! We were all put on a charge, and a few days later were tried by the lieutenant who was our platoon commander. Our sentence was a three Israeli Lira fine, to be deducted from our monthly salary of 12 Lira in three equal installments – hardly the transgression of a real rebel!

One of the men in our group was Neville. Neville was a product of the Betar movement in South Africa. Betar, to which Neville was a loyal devotee, is the youth movement affiliated with the right-wing Revisionist-Cherut (now Likud) political party, headed at that time by Menachem Begin, whose spiritual leader was Ze'ev Jabotinsky. Betar was the most militant, military-oriented of the Zionist youth movements, and service and obeying orders were important tenets of their education. Neville, like many of us, did not select this youth movement over that youth movement based on ideological grounds, but often on reasons as pedestrian as: "All the nice guys go there;" or, "They meet walking distance from my house;" or, "I hear their camps are more fun;" or "Such and such a girl I fancy goes there." Neville was by no stretch of the imagination an ideolog.

One of Neville's friends in the group told me the story that, when they were little boys in Betar, they used to go to the park and swing on the swings, and then jump off the swing while it was still moving. The idea of the game was to jump as far as possible, and this of course meant that the jump was quite scary. Neville was always scared to jump. His friends would say, "Come on, Neville, jump!" Neville continued swinging. "Come on, Neville, jump!" Neville continued swinging. "Come on, Neville, jump!" Neville continued swinging. Finally, getting nowhere, they would say, "Come on, Neville, jump for Israel!" and Neville would jump right away. Maybe he *was* a true ideolog after all.

Neville was a fine man, and was good at providing encouragement to others when the going got tough. On one occasion when we were on a particularly difficult route march Neville, realizing I was battling, came up alongside me and said, "David, you can do it. Fix your eyes on the shoulders of the guy in front of you and keep repeating, *Lema'an hamoledet hakol mutar*." (Translates roughly to: "Everything is achievable/permissible if it is for the homeland Israel)" I had a really good laugh over this, although Neville was quite serious in his advice. His Hebrew was virtually non-existent at that stage, and yet he said this to me in Hebrew because it was a kind of motto or mantra he had learned in the Betar movement in Johannesburg. He left Israel shortly after completing his service, and that is the last I ever heard of him.

Ivan was another of the characters. I've already mentioned how he almost got into serious trouble for mailing letters in a civilian box. But

Ivan was what we called a 'Histadrutnik' – a person who knew how to look after himself. Ivan somehow managed to get himself into the *Nachal* water polo team – I never did find out how he did it, especially as there was never any discussion or try-out for sports teams. Anyway, by dint of being on the team, he was given special leave after special leave to go to training sessions, and we were always green with envy. And when he did not have a training session he would contrive to kill off a close relative, whereupon it became, naturally, imperative for him to attend their funeral. Ivan's family was sorely depleted during those three and a half months.

Ivan was in his early-to-mid twenties when we were in basic training – substantially older than many of us. And his hair was already quite thin on top. One Friday night, some of our group got quite drunk, including Ivan. He was drunker than the rest. So a couple of soldiers grabbed clippers and shaved the top of Ivan's head, leaving him a rim of hair reminiscent of a monk. Little did they know that this was dead hair that they were removing, and that it would never grow back. Ivan being Ivan – incredibly good-natured – he took it very well. He, too, left Israel shortly after being discharged, and when I began writing this book I thought that he was still in South Africa. However, I learned recently from one of our group that he in fact came back to live in Israel just a few years ago where, sadly, he died.

Graham was another strange bird. He was one of the athletic types who had no difficulty with any of the physical challenges, and in fact was part of our group that went on to do Advanced Training, volunteering to become a paratrooper. I myself prefer using the steps to exit an airplane. At the time that we were doing our army service, the newly independent Congo was in the midst of the civil war ignited by the murder of its leader, Patrice Lumumba, about six months earlier. Well, word reached us that another South African, Mike Hoare, who was working as a mercenary for one of the militias in the Congo, was looking for volunteers who had been trained in the Israeli army, and was offering large salaries. Graham and a couple of other ex-South Africans signed up, and went from Israel straight into combat in the Congo for about six to eight months. I have not seen Graham since, but was told that he was almost killed in the fighting, but ultimately got out in one piece taking with him that huge salary, much of which he proceeded to splurge in England. That accomplished, he then returned to live in Israel.

One of the South Africans was named Hymie Kotzen. Every morning on the parade ground there was roll call, and we were supposed to remain quiet and serious and just shout out "Present, sir!" when our names were called. But when they got to Hymie, and the corporals daily called out "Kotching Heemie," we just cracked up. ('Kotching' in Yiddish means 'vomiting.') Hymie was less amused than the rest of us.

And then there was 'Sporting Sam.' He was a new immigrant from Romania who, probably due to an administrative error, ended up in this predominantly South African platoon. To this day, I have no idea what his name was, but we called him 'Sporting Sam' as he resembled a rotund cartoon character from the South African press. He must have had an awful time – he spoke no English and very little Hebrew, and I'm embarrassed to admit that we did precious little to make his life easier or more pleasant. One day, coming back from the showers in sandals, Sporting Sam stubbed his toe on a tent peg, and it was at that moment I heard him utter his first and only English swearword, "Barryscop!" – as it so happened, the name of another soldier serving with us. Somehow Sam had got it into his head that Barry Scop was a swearword, and that represented the sum total of the English that he learned during basic training.

Finally, let me tell you about Chalfon. We only knew him as Chalfon, not having the first clue as to whether this was his first or his last name. He, too, somehow fell into our platoon. I do not know much about Chalfon's background, but what I can tell you is that he was a new immigrant, like us. I think he was from North Africa, and he spoke Hebrew much more fluently than we did. In spite of our non-Hebrew conspiracy, we South Africans were in fact a very naïve bunch of kids. Not so Chalfon – he was always in trouble. He did not seem to take orders seriously. We were in awe of him because, unlike us, he did not seem to be at all afraid of our officers or of the authority they represented.

In the days after we were issued our rifles, our weapons instructors began to teach us how to take them apart. But there are different levels of 'taking apart,' and we were told in the firmest possible way that we were not to dismantle our rifles any further than we had been instructed to do. What we had been taught was to take the rifle apart just sufficiently to clean it and oil its working parts, *but to go no further.* There are many intricate springs, pins and screws in a rifle that only an armorer knows how to handle. Chalfon was bored on the Shabbat after we received our rifles, so he began to dismantle his rifle, and to dismantle his rifle, and to dismantle his rifle still further. But then came the task of putting it all together again, and he couldn't! The following morning, like every morning, we began the day with morning parade and inspection, which of course included inspection of our rifles. We were all standing on the parade ground with our rifles partially dismantled ready for our officers to inspect them and check that they were clean and oiled – all of us, that is, except for Chalfon – there he stood on the parade ground with the wooden butt of his rifle in one hand, and a tin of rifle oil filled with little screws, pins, springs and rivets in the other. Not all ranks present, particularly the more senior ones, were as amused as we were.

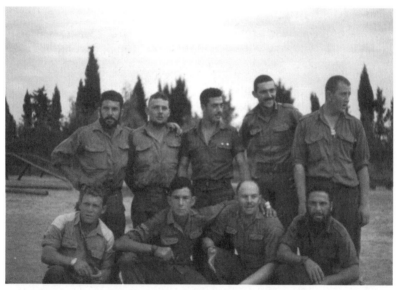

Some of the South Africans at the completion of basic training. I am in the front row, second from left, and next to me is a (balding) Ivan.

Much later on in basic training we spent a week out in the sand dunes doing field exercises. We had to take it in turns serving the food (such as it was), and in due course Chalfon's turn came to serve the monotonous breakfast which never varied – ever: very hard boiled eggs, a few olives, spring onions, bread and tea. Chalfon was sent to bring the eggs, and on his way back to where we used to sit in the sand and eat, he regrettably seized the opportunity to practice his soccer skills, tossing egg after egg into the air to see how far he could kick them. Unfortunately for him – and for us – one of our officers saw what was going on and, apart from Chalfon's personal punishment, from that day forth our platoon was given precisely the number of eggs to which it was entitled, but minus the 8 that Chalfon had employed as soccer balls. Strangely, we never got angry with him, principally because all these pranks he did diverted us, and we admired him for his bravado. I think we were also just slightly afraid of him. Although my theory was never put to the test, I sensed that this joker was an excellent soldier at heart, and the type of person one could rely on in combat.

My entire national service was carried out during a period of relative quiet and calm on Israel's borders. We were never involved in any combat, but we took part in complex maneuvers with live ammunition, and that, in and of itself, was realistic enough for my taste.

After completing basic training we were sent to work and do guard duty on a border kibbutz. However, when basic training ended in mid-November, two of us were chosen to stay on at the base for two weeks so that one of us could take a folk dancing and the other a singing course. The goal of these courses was for those who took them to go back to their groups on the kibbutz and to spearhead the social and cultural events of that group. Our South African group was far too macho for there to be any competition for these two slots. Who would ever want to take a singing or a dancing course? Only sissies would be interested. Norman asked to do the dancing course and I asked to do the singing course. In the event they actually proved to be quite exhausting – the dancing course even more so than the singing course. We began our days very early as always in the army, and I then spent something like 12 hours per day singing and learning new songs – or, as in Norman's case, dancing. Norman complained to me constantly how his muscles ached by the end of the day. Even learning new songs and singing them for that length of time a day, with no let-up even for Shabbat, was very tiring, and somehow all the fun was drained out of it. The army did have a knack for this sort of stupidity.

At this point we were the 'vatikim' (old-timers) on the base – the ones who had been there for over three months, who had completed basic training, and who were doing something more appealing than what most of the other people, who were new recruits, were doing.

Being the *vatikim*, we were also quite used to the base's antiquated toilets, unique constructions of British origin since the whole army base, including the toilets, had been built by the British during the pre-1948 Mandate, and so could not be described as state of the art. The toilets took the form of a very deep pit, over which the British had built a huge circular concrete slab to the height of a chair, with eight slots carved out so that eight of us sat on the slab over the slot at once. Enough said. You can imagine that entering these toilets was quite a sight – eight men, pants around their ankles, sitting in a circle facing outwards, backs to each other, and all chatting and laughing together – sort of like the petals of a flower.

On the Friday night during the singing/dancing course, Norman and I were walking past the toilets when we heard a commotion going on. We went to see what was happening, only to learn that one of the new recruits had let his wallet with all his money and his documents fall out of his pants' pocket into the pit! This was a very serious matter. There were no electric lights in that part of the base, so what the soldiers were doing was dangling a lantern from a rope down into the pit from the adjacent slot, and then lowering another rope with a piece of hook-shaped wire at the end from the luckless wallet owner's slot. This was an extremely tricky maneuver, needless to say, as that revolting pit must have been at least 20 feet deep. Quite a crowd had gathered in and around the toilet, and much advice was proffered and many jokes cracked. Believe it or not, they managed to harpoon the wallet and then to retrieve it. I gave them full marks for their ingenuity as well as the strength of their stomachs. Above all, though, this episode is ultimate proof of the power of Israeli bureaucracy at that time, since the difficulties involved in trying to harpoon all the lost documents that must have been in that wallet out of a thirty-year old cesspit paled besides those that would have been involved in endeavoring to have them officially replaced.

Basic training lasted three and a half months. When I'd completed it I was as slim and as fit as I have ever been. I entered the army weighing 195 lbs., and left weighing 160 and feeling wonderful.

The rest of my army service was spent on two different border kibbutzim. The first was Kibbutz Gesher on the Jordanian border, on the Jordan River in the Beit She'an Valley, just south of the Sea of Galilee. Our task was to work on the kibbutz alongside the kibbutzniks and also to provide military reinforcement to the kibbutz both in terms of general guard duty as well as in times of emergency.

We were still soldiers, wore uniform, and had some sort of inspection of our living quarters and equipment daily. However, we were living, working, and interacting with the civilian population of the kibbutz. We lived in huts that belonged to the kibbutz, but which were no longer used by them. We also ate in the communal dining room with the kibbutz members, were allowed to attend the weekly movie with them, and unless we had some military duties were at liberty to socialize with them. The women who had been in our group rejoined us at this point, and lived and worked on the kibbutz for the remainder of their service.

Based on what I had learned in Habonim, I knew that there was a tradition for kibbutz families to 'adopt' volunteers or soldiers living on their kibbutz. This meant that you were assigned to the family who had adopted you, and you spent every afternoon after work and a siesta with them having tea and socializing, very often went with them to the communal dining room for supper, and sat with them at all parties, festivals, and other gatherings.

Arriving two weeks after everybody else because of the singing course, I was shocked and disappointed to learn that nothing had been done abut adopting us. So I moved into action immediately and set up adoptions for all members of our group who were interested, and was myself adopted by Pnina and Ya'akov. They and their children welcomed me warmly into their family, and I really loved being with them. In fact, I told them several times that on completion of my university studies I would return to live on the kibbutz, but they knew better and just smiled whimsically and said that, once I left the kibbutz, I would never return. And they were right.

We were required to work a full day, and every evening we were assigned our work for the next day. Much of it was seasonal agricultural work, hard physically and monotonous. Many of the people who served with me hated the work. I, by chance, was placed early on to work in the fish ponds – of which this kibbutz had many, each the size of a football field, where they raised carp for marketing. This was hard labor, as we often had to trudge through thick mud dragging huge fish nets filled with hundreds of fully grown carp, a truly Sisyphean task. When there was a shipment of fish to be sent to market we had to work extra hours, yet at the same time it was strangely satisfying work and we worked well as a team. And because I enjoyed the work I found that I worked well, so was assigned to work in the fish ponds almost the entire time I was stationed at Kibbutz Gesher.

The military demands placed on us were not extensive, which suited me perfectly. Moreover, the security situation was quiet during that period (late 1961 – early 1962), the only really serious incident while we were at Gesher being the battle which took place at Nuqueib, east of the Sea of Galilee. Like all units in the north of the country we were put on high alert, but we were not actually involved in the fighting, although we were close enough to be able to hear the shells exploding. In the great scheme of things this was really little more than a border skirmish, but given that it was the only major incident that occurred during my national service, it took on a greater meaning for me. It was largely small arms infantry combat, and nothing of political or strategic significance came out of it. Sadly, as always, there were losses on both sides.

The buildings of Kibbutz Gesher are situated about half a kilometer west of the Jordan River, with the fields stretching down to the very banks of the river – the international border with Jordan. 'Gesher' means 'bridge,' and the kibbutz took its name from a bridge over the

Jordan that had been built by the British to carry the railway line from Haifa to Damascus, but which had been blown up in the middle during the War of Independence. We could see the Jordanian soldiers on the east side of the river, but they ignored us unless we actually walked onto what remained of the bridge. At that moment they would rush down to their side of the narrow river, crouch down and aim their rifles at us, remaining in the firing position until we turned around and walked back westwards and off the bridge. We used to do this just for fun.

Pnina and Ya'akov, my adoptive family on the kibbutz, treated me like their son, or at least like a close cousin from overseas. I went to their room for tea every afternoon, and from there to the communal dining room for supper, where I sat with them. They did not speak very good English, and this gave me a perfect opportunity to practice my Hebrew – the conspiracy of ignorance having long since ceased to exist.

Pnina and Ya'akov even invited my parents to come up to the kibbutz for a weekend as their guests, a typically generous gesture that delighted us all. My parents, as new immigrants, were entitled for a limited period to import one car duty free, a significant concession which meant that they had to pay a little less than 50% of the usual price in Israel. As a result, most immigrants were prepared to borrow the money in order to be able to acquire a car on such advantageous terms even when, like my parents, they strictly speaking could not afford it. My parents, as a result, had just bought a brand new Morris Mini Minor, of which they were very proud, and it was in this gleaming new purchase that they drove up to the Galilee. I decided to give them a little surprise while we were touring the kibbutz, so I told them to stay where they were while I, in my uniform, walked onto the bridge. Like clockwork, two Jordanian soldiers came down to their side of the bridge, aimed their rifles at me and waited until I walked away before standing easy. My mother, in particular, was extremely upset. At the time I could not understand why my parents were not amused, but as I write this I am almost ten years older than they were then, and can now clearly see that what I did was really neither very clever nor very amusing.

I was at Kibbutz Gesher from the end of November, 1961, until the middle of May the following year. During that period my parents' *ulpan* came to an end, and they moved to Jerusalem and began their jobs. They had, as immigrants, been eligible to apply for subsidized housing through the Jewish Agency, and had been promised a two-bedroom apartment in a building that was still under construction. In the meantime, they were allowed to live in a hostel called 'The Anglo-Saxon Hostel' in the Jerusalem suburb of Rasco. This was an exceptionally dreary boarding house owned by the Jewish Agency, and its name belies its appearance. In fact, it was quite awful. The saving grace was that it was temporary and it was very cheap.

In those days I wore glasses most, but not all, of the time. During basic training, while doing an exercise of carrying wounded on our shoulders, my glasses got kicked out of my shirt pocket and lost. I was, however, most impressed to learn that the army would replace them for me free of charge. Unfortunately I was to learn later that there was a small catch to the army's apparent generosity.

It came about in this way. While I was at Kibbutz Gesher, I managed to lose my glasses for a second time. I was completely unconcerned, confident that the army would again replace them for me *gratis*. But what I did not know was that on this occasion, because the *army* had supplied the glasses the previous time, what I had lost was not personal but military property, thereby making me culpable of a military offence. Having applied for new glasses, I was shocked to be informed that I was to report to the base which served as our unit's headquarters – for a military trial! The charge? Loss of military equipment. I was absolutely appalled, but had had no choice but to set off and report to the base in question. On arrival, I was treated like any accused awaiting trial, and was placed with a group of soldiers charged with (at least in my opinion) much more serious offences. While in my head I knew how idiotic this was, in my heart I was quite scared, and did not enjoy being barked at by the sergeant major in question, being marched into the courtroom and being addressed and referred to as 'the accused.'

I explained how I had lost my glasses, and to my intense relief was acquitted and given permission to replace them once again at the army's expense. From then on I was extremely careful with them, wearing them all the time, as indeed I have done ever since.

A month before I left Kibbutz Gesher my brother, Steve, arrived in Israel – he had duly completed an additional year at university in South Africa and, according to plan, had immigrated. I applied for special leave to go and meet him, and was granted five days. He went directly to my parents' home in Rasco, 'The Anglo-Saxon Hostel.' This dingy, uninviting building was heated with kerosene heaters which, although relatively effective, made the place reek of kerosene, and to this day, whenever I happen to be in that suburb, all I can think of is that awful smell.

My parents had rented an additional room for Steve, which I shared when I was on leave. After I had been there for about two days, I came down with a severe case of chicken pox, became really sick and ran a high fever. There was no way I could return to the kibbutz on the appointed day. We notified the military authorities, and they granted me a couple of extra weeks at home until I was fully recovered. I was visited by a military doctor who told me that, to reduce the itching, I should daub the spots with 'brilliant green.' Brilliant green, as its name implies, is iodine colored bright green, and is used extensively in Israel to clean and disinfect wounds. The spots were extremely itchy, and one night Steve came back after going out for the evening to find that I had painted my entire face green in the hope of getting some relief. Instead of being sympathetic, he just burst out laughing. This was my first encounter with the magic of military medicine. The doctor I saw while I was still covered with spots decided that the spots were not just chicken pox, and sent me to see a dermatologist. I was delighted, as this took a couple of days and thereby prolonged my time with my family. When the dermatologist examined me he, of course, identified my spots as nothing more than the common or garden brand of chicken pox spots – even I, a not-yet-medic, could have told him that, but I was not complaining at being able to enjoy extra days of leave. But this additional medical leave carried with it a terrible price.

On my return to the kibbutz, I learned that my trials at the hands of military justice were by no means over. I was again ordered to report to headquarters the following week for yet another trial. I was thunderstruck! I had done nothing wrong. I asked what the charge was, and was told that while I was away, enjoying my medically extended leave, a high ranking armorer had come to inspect every soldier's rifle – including the rifles of those of us who were away – stored securely in the armory under the care of our unit armorer. And he had found rust in my rifle – a very serious offence in *Tzahal*. I tried to protest that it was not my responsibility as I had been away ill. On the contrary, I was told, it was very much my fault, and that not only had I to attend the trial but also to take every piece of military equipment in my possession with me so that it could be placed in storage should I be sentenced to a lengthy term in military prison. This alarmed me greatly, and what is more I had a ton of equipment, including bedding, and no transportation was provided to take the accused to their trials. I don't know how I managed it, but I lugged all the equipment up to the main road and from there hitchhiked a ride to the base.

Once again, I was marched briskly into the courtroom, and again pleaded my case as best I could in my broken Hebrew. The presiding officer listened attentively to me, and then began to speak:

"This is a very serious offence. You do not treat your rifle with the care that *Tzahal* demands. Now, I have studied your file and I see that you are a good and conscientious soldier … " It was beginning to sound good, but then he continued: "And because of that, I have decided that you have to learn your lesson, and I am therefore sentencing you to military prison for thirty days…"

I could not believe my ears! I was going to jail! I was both upset and badly frightened. I just stood there, frozen. And then, after what seemed like an eternity, he added, "suspended for six months." I heaved a sigh of relief. A suspended sentence means that there is this threat of the punishment hanging over you, in my case for six months, and if there is any other offence during that time, then the prison sentence is actuated. If not, then it is wiped from your record after the stipulated six months. I literally skipped back to the road to hitchhike back to the kibbutz, and never complained one bit about the weight of the equipment. I resolved only that for the next six months my rifle would always be *very* well oiled. In retrospect, I've discovered that it was wrong for me to have been put on trial; rather, it was the armorer who was responsible for my rifle during that period; but at the time I did not know better, and the armorer was certainly not inclined to enlighten me.

In mid-May, those of us who did not opt for advanced training and parachuting were transferred to a different kibbutz, Lehavot Habashan, on the Syrian border at the foot of the Golan Heights. This, too, was an agreeable experience – in fact, it was an even nicer kibbutz than Gesher, despite the somewhat nerve-wracking guard duty we had to do under the very noses of the Syrians. Luckily for me, this period passed uneventfully, although Lehavot Habashan and those in the vicinity were always vulnerable to attack from the high ground held by the Syrians directly above them.

On Kibbutz Lehavot Habashan I requested to work in their fish ponds, given my 'vast' experience at Kibbutz Gesher, and as at Gesher I worked there almost the entire time. I was once again adopted by a family, and once again loved the experience.

While on the kibbutz, I became friendly with Yossie, a kibbutz member in his thirties, originally from Turkey. Yossie told me that he was teaching himself English, and asked me if I would tutor him. I had never tutored anyone in my life, and had no idea that teaching English as a Foreign Language was to become my lifelong career, but the idea appealed to me and I agreed. I'd already decided that I wanted to be a teacher rather than an agronomist, so I decided to give it a try. The officer in charge of us, Amir, was impressed that I would be tutoring, and immediately exempted me from our weekly fitness class, which included a lengthy run. What a great deal!

And so began my first teaching experience, and one that does not feature on my *curriculum vitae*. When we sat down to our first lesson, Yossie told me that he had been working, on his own, from an English grammar textbook. I asked him what he had learned, and this is what he said, *verbatim*:

Singular:	Plural:
Ani ochel – I eat	*Anachnu ochlim* – we eat
Ata ochel – you eat	*Atem ochlim* – you (plural) eat
Hu ochel – he eats	*Heym ochlim* – they (masculine) eat
Hi ochelet – she eats	*Heyn ochlot* – "chey" (feminine) eat

When I asked him about "chey eat" he explained: *Heym ochlim* is "they (plural, masculine) eat," and *Heyn ochlot* is "they (plural, feminine) eat," and so this corresponded to "they" and "chey" for the masculine and feminine forms in his English. In my linguistics studies, I subsequently learned how hard it is for second language learners when they are confronted by a gap in English where there is a special form in their own first language. I never did find out where he got the "chey" from, but it certainly was a good idea, and ever since I have been tempted to say things like: "Look at the boys. They are playing football." "Look at the girls. Chey are playing tennis."

Just around the time I moved to Kibbutz Lehavot Habashan, my parents moved into their apartment. It was tiny, and on the fourth floor – sixty four steps up and no elevator – but it was home! I will never forget the first leave I had after they moved in. I walked into the living-room/dining area, and there were all sorts of familiar items from our home in Johannesburg: the carpet, the pictures, ornaments, the ash-trays, the silver cigarette lighter, the cigarette box, the cutlery and crockery, and more. My mother had managed to transform this tiny, anonymous apartment into a real home for us.

As the time ticked by, I realized that I was due to be discharged just a few weeks after the start of the academic year at university. I mentioned this to Amir, the officer in charge of us on the kibbutz, and he immediately said I should write a letter requesting an early discharge so as not to lose the academic year – in fact, he wrote the letter for me, and appended his recommendation. This was a time when only a small proportion of Israel's population attended university, and Amir was clearly taken with the idea that one of his soldiers should be going to university. It just so happened that Amir and I worked together in the fish ponds and one day, as we were trudging back from work, exhausted, we stopped at the dining room to get something to drink, and I saw there was a letter for me – lo and behold, it was an official letter granting me the early discharge. I immediately told Amir as we continued walking up to our rooms, and his response was "Don't slouch – stand up straight like a student!" I think that is the most respect I have ever received for being a student or an academic. No one before or since has ever called on me to deport myself "as a student." Nor, for that matter, as a professor. I was amused by Amir's response because, having grown up in privileged white South African society, I had always assumed that I would in any case automatically be going to university.

I was discharged in mid October of that year, and was now not only a civilian but also a "miluimnik" – a reservist. All able-bodied Israelis, when they complete their army service, automatically go into *miluim*, and are then called up on a regular basis for training and active service. And I remained a *miluimnik* for as long as I lived in Israel.

I ended my compulsory national service as a trained, yet unspecialized soldier – a rifleman, and was placed in a reserve infantry unit. I remained in this unit, Company 161 of the Jerusalem Brigade, until 1977, a period which straddled both the Six Day and the Yom Kippur Wars. We were a front-line combat unit, and our reserve duty was always a mix of refresher exercises with maneuvers and of active service on the border. Once I became a medic, there were often an additional few days of refresher training in First Aid. After 1967, our *miluim* frequently included exchanges of fire, injury and even the death of some members of our unit. So if I were to sum up what *miluim* was like for me, I'd describe it as either boring, physically taxing or dangerous, or some mix of these three undesirable elements.

Serving as a *miluimnik* was a new experience, the culture of *miluim* being quite different from what I had known as a national serviceman. Literally everybody up to the rank of battalion commander was a *miluimnik*, and discipline was there, not for its own sake, but to ensure that what needed to be done, however unpleasant or dangerous it might be, was done. There was no saluting or referring to an officer by rank or title – we just used first names. This is not to suggest that there was no respect for rank or for the authority that it carried, because in that respect it was just like any other army, except that the external trappings were not present. But we all knew precisely who was who, and an order was an order. For example, our battalion commander at the time of the Six Day War was named Asher, and we all addressed him as Asher, but he was still very much the battalion commander. Officers from the rank of lieutenant and upwards tended to wear their rank, but the rest of us did not – after all, if someone of the rank of sergeant had some special responsibilities in the platoon, we all knew who he was, so there was no need for the stripes. This was not an attempt at creating an army of 'equals' – there was no Communist ideology – as *Tzahal* is a regular army with all the ranks and authority that this implies. The difference is that the lower ranks usually do not bother to wear their stripes.

Another unique feature of *miluim* units was the huge disparity in age between the soldiers. At that time, soldiers remained in a front line unit like ours until the age of thirty-nine, and were then moved to a less active unit. I was not yet twenty when I joined my unit, and there were people like Avraham, aged thirty nine, serving with me, who had been in the unit since the early 1950s. At the time, I thought he was really old. Although today it seems young to me, it is old for the kind of physical demands placed on an infantryman.

The backgrounds of the people I served with were also extremely varied. Avraham, as it so happens, was an unskilled worker at the Friedman factory where my father worked. Many of the reservists were immigrants from North African and Arab countries, and the *lingua franca* of the unit was Arabic and not Hebrew; knowing that I did not speak Arabic, they would considerately change over to Hebrew for my sake whenever I was present. There were laborers in the building industry, truck drivers, owners of vegetable stalls in the market, civil servants, academics and more. I personally have never had any difficulty getting along with people, and certainly had none with everybody in the unit regardless of their background. In fact, as part of my idealistic view of Israel, I found this to be one of the more positive and exciting aspects of Israeli society. This was not true for everyone. For example, at one point a new soldier, Aaron, joined our platoon. I happened to know him from Jerusalem, where he worked as a middle-level civil servant in the Ministry of Tourism where my mother worked. He did not hold a very important position – I can vouch for that. However, he arrived with a massive chip on his shoulder, and began treating his comrades as if they were stupid and inferior to him. It was ugly. Then, suddenly, without a word ever being said about Aaron's behavior or what to do about it, within a few days the platoon began to ostracize him. No one opened conversations with him; no one sat with him at meals – in short, as the British say, he was 'sent to Coventry.' I truly believe that he deserved this treatment, and I had no sympathy for him. In due course he was placed in another unit; I do hope that he had learned something while in our platoon, but I am highly doubtful.

I came 'home' to my new Israeli civilian world: to my parents, to the new apartment, to sharing a room once again with Steve – a very *alt-neu* (old-new) feeling. There were only a few weeks remaining before the university year began, and I had quite a lot to do to get ready. I registered in the B.A. program in the double majors of General History (as opposed to Jewish History, which was a separate department) and English Literature. At that time at the Hebrew University you had to have two majors, and mine were chosen with a view to utilizing them both in my career as a teacher. As my life has unfolded and my likes and dislikes for different disciplines developed, I have hardly ever worked as a History teacher, except for a brief period in 1977 when I was supply teaching. Moreover, by the time I was two-thirds of the way through my B.A., I knew that my real interest was Applied Linguistics – Linguistic theory as it applies to Second Language Acquisition and Pedagogy.

Steve was also registered to do a B.A., majoring in Political Science and English Literature, so that we had several classes together, which was quite a strange experience for the 'little brother.' The academic year was divided into trimesters, and by half way through the first trimester I had noticed and become interested in a beautiful, tall girl from England who was in several of my English classes. Her name was Jennifer (Jenny), and I soon found out that she was not from England at all, but from Durban, South Africa. She and her mother and sister, Beverley, had made Aliyah in February of that year, joining her brother, Leon, who was already in Israel. On December 16, 1962, I invited her out on a date, and from that day to this we have never gone out with anyone else. We announced our engagement in October of the following year, and married in Jerusalem a year later on December 31, four months before my twenty first birthday. Jenny, too, was majoring in English Literature (and Psychology), and so she sat between Steve and me in several courses over the next two and a half years. Some of our fellow students in the English Department monitored the development of our romance, and many years later we were to become friendly with Puah, who was a student at the same time, and who informed us that not only had we all been in class together, but she had even written a short story about our romance as she tracked it in the English Department.

Steve, for his part, had come to Israel leaving his girlfriend, Ami, in South Africa. They had met at Habonim camp, and a serious relationship had begun there and then. Ami was finishing high school at that stage, and in January, 1963, she arrived in Israel on the same one year youth leadership program that Steve had been on when he first arrived in Israel.

My mother had always argued that her home had 'rubber walls,' and that everyone was welcome. Her theory was put to the test that year: Jenny and I began going out in earnest in December, while she was living in university residence since her mother lived in Givatayim, near Tel Aviv. What happened in reality is that, virtually every night, Jenny would come to us for supper, and more often than not she would sleep over on a camp bed in the living room. And then Ami arrived, and whenever she had a night off on her course, she too ate with us and slept over – also on a camp bed in the living room. In addition to the weekday visitors, Jenny's mother and sister, Beverley, used to come to Jerusalem often, and they were always welcome at my parents' home. The two sets of parents grew extremely close, and after we were married either my parents went to Givatayim to spend the weekend with my mother-in-law, or she came up to Jerusalem. Beverley, for her part, became closely attached to my parents, and to this day talks of her very deep love for them.

My parents never complained, although it must have been quite an imposition on them. Not only did they have one or two people sleeping in their living room almost nightly, but to get from their bedroom to the kitchen they had to pass through that living room/dining area, and many times they crept through and quietly ate their breakfast there while Jenny and Ami slept. What is more, they were living on the tightest of budgets, and two extra mouths over and above our regular four meant a not insignificant additional cost.

Steve's and Ami's relationship blossomed. During the following year they became engaged, and were married in Johannesburg in December, 1965. On completion of his degree, a year later, Steve was appointed as an educational officer to the Zionist movement in South Africa, working mainly with Jewish university students, and they returned to Johannesburg where they worked until the middle of 1969, at which time they returned to Israel.

I began my undergraduate studies in November, and it was all very well being a student, but I was also *a miluimnik*, liable for military service every year. This invariably conflicted with my studies. If call up came during term-time, then we were expected to go and make up what we missed, and it was rare that we would succeed in being released on the grounds of missing class. Mine was not an exceptional situation – nor is it even today – and the professors were supposed to help you make up what you had missed, and were required to give you an extension on assignments due. This was officially also the policy when it came to exams – you were supposed to go to *miluim*, and a special sitting of the exam would be arranged for you. However, when the service conflicted with exams, the army was more understanding, and you were entitled to apply to a special army committee for a deferment of service, and wherever possible this was granted.

My first *miluim* was in the spring of 1963. Serving together is a great leveler, with people from all walks of life thrown together every few months in the most difficult of circumstances, and having to help each other to cope (and to survive). It does not take long for a special camaraderie to develop among the men, even though they may have absolutely nothing in common in civilian life, so that over the years I grew really close with many of the other reservists.

The most important way in which *Tzahal* leveled society was that there was truly equal opportunity, and one's origin or first language or social status did not play any part in who rose through the ranks. It would be naïve of me to pretend that the social stratification of Israeli society with Ashkenazi Jews (Jews of Eastern European origin) above Sephardic Jews (Jews from North Africa and the Arab world) did not penetrate into the military. It did and, needless to say, soldiers who came from families that had had more opportunities for education and betterment in their civilian lives often had the edge in the army as well. However, anyone in the army who had the ability and the desire to advance could do so.

Another way in which *Tzahal* served as a leveler was with regard to language. Hebrew was the language of the army, and gradually over my years in *miluim*, I saw the disappearance of Arabic and other foreign languages in the day to day conversation of virtually everyone.

There were wonderfully anomalous situations that *Tzahal* created, and which I loved. For example, my company sergeant major – a man who wielded a fair amount of power over us privates – worked in civilian life for the Jerusalem Municipality, and his job was to clear blocked sewers. I often would see him about to disappear down a manhole as I drove past *en route* to the university, and we would call out a friendly hello to each other. Another of my comrades in the platoon was an usher at one of the downtown movie theaters, and he would show us to our seats whenever we went to that cinema. Yet another delicious example of all of this leveling process was one I encountered at the time of the Yom Kippur War, at which point I was serving as a medic in the Battalion Aid Station (*ta'agad*), alongside a team of *chovshim* (medics) and a doctor. Our battalion doctor was a specialist physician working at Hadassah, Jerusalem's largest hospital. He, in turn reported to the brigade doctor, who was one rank higher than him in the military, but in civilian life the brigade doctor, by chance in the same specialty area as our battalion doctor, reported to him.

In 1964, the army realized that I did not have a 'military profession'

– some more specialized training – and I began getting call ups to take specialized courses. The courses often conflicted with university examinations, and on two occasions when that occurred the army's special committee excused me from taking the course. The first time, but for the examination, I would have become a sapper – a combat soldier who lays, detonates, and dismantles mines and bombs. This is a particularly unpopular and dangerous job, and I was delighted that an exam saved me from becoming a sapper. The second time it was a mortar course from which my academic studies saved me – a little better, but again, not something I particularly relished. But then none of the army's jobs greatly appealed to me, and I was reconciled to the fact that I would not be thrilled whatever the course. Finally, in the summer of 1964, I was called to a 'chovesh kravi' ('combat medic') course and, since this did not conflict with any of my exams, I had no excuse and no choice. I had received an order to take this course, that was simply not negotiable, so off I went. So much for career counseling, army-style.

I have always had an interest in medicine, and the prospect of being a medic was most appealing – certainly a lot more so than being a sapper, a mortar man, or many other things. Mind you, I had no idea what being a medic in the infantry really meant. What I did know was that being a *chovesh kravi* did not mean that I would be wearing a white coat with a stethoscope slung around my neck, assisting a doctor in some field hospital stationed safely to the rear. I was to learn many, many years later that that was, indeed, the perception of my children. I, however, had had the opportunity of seeing the medics in my own infantry unit, and knew that they were very much a part of the unit, and that they functioned just like the rest of the soldiers unless or until there was an injury requiring their attention.

In spite of my interest in the field of medicine, I'd been warned by many people in my unit that this was a terrible branch of the military in which to serve. Common wisdom had it that being a *chovesh* in a combat unit was unattractive for a large number of reasons: it is gory and revolting dealing with the injured, the dead and the dying, particularly on the battlefield, as *chovshim* of my rank would be doing. Second, there is a chronic shortage of *chovshim* in *Tzahal*, so *chovshim* find themselves doing the maximum amount of reserve duty, and if by chance their unit is inactive at any point, the army makes sure that the *chovesh* is seconded to another unit to fill the ever-present shortage. Moreover, whereas riflemen moved out of a front-line combat unit at age 39, *chovshim* were kept in these units until the age of 41. *Chovshim* were also expected to run and train with the regular riflemen, the only difference being that you carried a huge amount of medical supplies and equipment plus a stretcher, as well as your own rifle and ammunition. In addition, *chovshim* were called up for about three additional days prior to the arrival of the riflemen, so as to have a refresher course in First Aid. To cap it all, being a *chovesh* was, in military circles, a low prestige branch of the army. What is more, being a *chovesh* in the infantry is dangerous: you're right up there in the front with the platoon commander and the radio operator, prime targets for the enemy, who understood only too well that knocking out any one of us would severely hamper the unit's effectiveness.

Above all, there was the factor that I was to find out – but only years later when I wanted a transfer – that "once a *chovesh*, always a *chovesh*," meaning that it was next to impossible to be reassigned out of this job. It came about in this way. It happened that in the 1970's the army began using language laboratories for some of its teaching, and at the time I was Director of Language Laboratories at the Hebrew University. One day, I was contacted by some high ranking officer in the regular army asking whether I would agree to being transferred from the combat unit I was in to the educational unit, so that I could help them with their language laboratory. My heart leapt with delight – finally I was getting out of the front line and would be doing my *miluim* in an office, probably not even having to sleep away from home. I told him I was more than ready to make the move. He told me that he would make the necessary arrangements and get back to me. Many weeks passed, and then he called me:

"I have bad news. We need you, but you are not being transferred to us."

"What happened?" I asked, unable to disguise my disappointment.

"When I spoke to your Brigade Commander to arrange the transfer, he immediately agreed, on condition that I send him a replacement combat medic."

And that was the end of that.

But, in spite of all the negatives, on the other side of the argument were two compelling points. First, I felt that this was the one arm of the military in which the goal was not to kill or to maim, but to help and to heal, a view that agreed well with my latent pacifistic sympathies. And the other even more compelling argument was that I had no choice – I had received an order to take this course, and that was not negotiable.

The course took place in the summer of 1964. That was the summer that preceded my first teaching job and Jenny's and my wedding. The negative attitude of the course members was evident from the day the course began – more than half of the people called up with me for the course tried to get out of it, (unsuccessfully, I should add), and almost every one of us, whether we liked it or not, became combat medics. We qualified as platoon medics, which was the lowest rank within the medical hierarchy. Our training was very much field first aid, but in 1967 I was to find out that we certainly had learned enough to cover most emergencies.

One of the oddest incidents of the whole course involved one of our instructors, a sergeant named Teddy. He was a short, stocky, serious, and intensely pompous man. It is interesting that in that kind of setting, once the group perceives that an officer or instructor is too serious or 'square,' they will find ways to bug him, and we did. Well, it fell to Teddy to teach us how to lift and carry wounded soldiers without stretchers – a skill I'd need many times in the years to come. Teddy looked over the group, and pointed to me, the largest specimen, and told me to lie down on the ground so that he could demonstrate. I said to him that I was much too heavy for him to lift. "Shut up and lie down; and lie limp – don't try and help me!" Like a good soldier, I did what he told me, and with much huffing and puffing he managed to lift me across his shoulders and to run about 110 metres. This was no small feat, as there was a substantial difference between our sizes and weights. The next day Teddy was not with us, nor the next day, nor the day after that. We could no longer assume that he was on leave, so we asked where he was, and were informed that he was in hospital with a slipped disc.

What being a platoon medic meant was that we would be designated as the medic responsible for one platoon (about 25 soldiers), and would be with these men as they advanced. The plan was that there was also a company medic, to whom we, the platoon medics, reported, and above him was the *ta'agad* – the furthermost forward position where there was a doctor, and with him a team of more highly trained *chovshim*. We were not allowed to move back from the front line even to evacuate wounded – we had to get riflemen to do that, and they would evacuate the wounded back to the *ta-agad*. The *ta'agad* team would attend to and stabilize the wounded, and then send them back to their units or evacuate them as the doctor decided. And then behind the *ta'agad* was a field hospital. The field hospital is the equivalent of the United States' M*A*S*H unit. In other words, I was right at the front, two steps in front of the M*A*S*H unit so well popularized on television.

Between the end of the course in 1964 and the outbreak of the Six Day War in 1967 I did a substantial amount of *miluim*. However these were quiet times, and I functioned as I always had – as a rifleman who was also the platoon medic, the only difference being the extra equipment I had to carry. Throughout the period of my *miluim* until the outbreak of the Six Day War we saw no combat, did not do much active service on the border, and our *miluim* consisted mainly of refresher days in First Aid, field exercises and occasional spells of guard duty at settlements near the border. And, true to what I'd been told we, the *chovshim*, were indeed treated with scant respect, and I might even say with some disdain. All this was to change dramatically within two hours of the outbreak of the Six Day War.

So that is how I came to find myself serving in the front lines, on June 5, 1967, under mortar fire from the Jordanians, as a combat medic in an infantry unit in the Six Day War.

Part II

THE SIX DAY WAR

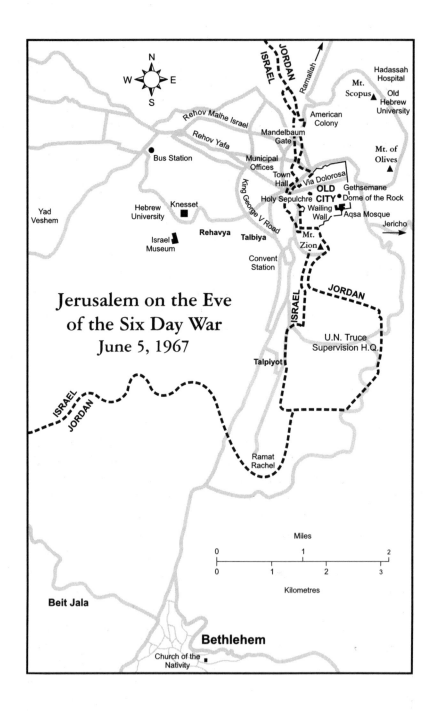

How does one explain an event as momentous as the Six Day War, and what it felt like to be a simple civilian-cum-soldier caught up in it? This little book does not attempt anything so ambitious. All I've tried to do is to describe some of the unique moments *I* experienced – some sad, some uplifting, some even funny.

From my perspective, it all began on Yom Ha'Atzma'ut (Independence Day) on May 15, 1967. By then, Jenny and I had been married for two and a half years, but we did not have any children yet. A year earlier we had managed to purchase a modest, very small apartment on Nili Street, and were intensely proud of our first home. We had both graduated with our B.A.s and, in addition, I had completed a graduate teaching diploma, qualifying me as a high school teacher of English (as a foreign language) and History. Jenny was working at the Jewish National and University Library at the Hebrew University, and I was teaching English at the Hebrew University Secondary School, adjacent to the university campus at Givat Ram. At that time, this was the only university campus in Jerusalem, since the Mount Scopus campus lay outside the 1949 armistice lines, so that although it was still recognized as sovereign Israeli territory, it was only accessible to Israeli police, who were taken through Jordanian territory to guard it. There was no way it could be used as a university.

My parents were still in the same jobs and had settled into a routine in their new lives in Jerusalem. They worked long hours, six days a week, and were really too tired to do much else during the week. Their lifestyle was modest, as their circumstances did not permit them the luxuries that make life that much easier, such as a person to clean the apartment, or buying prepared foods. They had made a small number of friends, but most of their relaxation time was spent with Jenny and me and our friends, most of whom regarded them as loving, surrogate parents. Steve and Ami were still in Johannesburg, Steve still working for the Zionist movement.

In those days, the Independence Day celebrations always ended after sunset with the annual Israeli Song Contest. This was a big event, and every year we would settle down in our living room in front of the radio to listen to the songs – at that time Israel did not have television. This contest was not only a very enjoyable evening's entertainment, but it gave us a chance to hear all the new songs which were destined to become the hits of the coming year. In later years, the winning song went on to be Israel's entry in the Eurovision Song Contest.

In addition to the songs entered in the contest, one song had been commissioned by the Mayor of Jerusalem, Teddy Kollek, and it was to receive its maiden airing mid-way through the contest. That song was *Yerushalayim Shel Zahav* (*Jerusalem of Gold*), written by Naomi Shemer and sung by Shuli Natan. This was to become as close as any song could come to being a second anthem, inextricably linked to the war that was only three weeks away, although none of us then could foresee that. It has a hauntingly beautiful melody, with even more haunting lyrics. It is a song about 'golden Jerusalem' and our yearning to return to the markets and streets of the Old City, to the Western Wall and the Temple Mount, all of which had been held by Jordan since the 1948 War of Independence and which were, therefore, in enemy territory:

JERUSALEM OF GOLD

The mountain air is clear as water
The scent of pines around
Is carried on the breeze of twilight
And tinkling bells resound.

The trees and stones there softly slumber,
A dream enfolds them all.
So solitary lies the city,
And at its heart – a wall.

Chorus

Oh, Jerusalem of gold, and of light and of bronze,
I am the lute for all your songs.

The wells ran dry of all their water,
Forlorn the market square,
The Temple Mount dark and deserted,
In the Old City there.

And in the caverns in the mountain,
The winds howl to and fro,
And no-one takes the Dead Sea highway,
That leads through Jericho.

Chorus

But as I sing to you, my city,
And you with crowns adorn,
I am the least of all your children,
Of all the poets born.

Your name will scorch my lips for ever,
Like a seraph's kiss, I'm told,
If I forget thee, golden city,
Jerusalem of gold.

Chorus

As I'd only come to Israel in 1961, 'my' Jerusalem consisted of West Jerusalem, with the Old City, the Western Wall, The Mount of Olives, The Hebrew University on Mount Scopus, Augusta Victoria Hospital, Bethlehem and more, merely places we knew about and tried to squint at from strategic observation points, but access to which was denied us. Without any knowledge of its prophetic nature, simply because of the beauty of its words and melody, *Yerushalayim Shel Zahav* became an instant hit. And, in fact, it has subsequently been judged the number one hit of all time in Israel.

Three days later, on May 18, U Thant, Secretary General of the United Nations, at President Gamal Abdul Nasser of Egypt's request, announced that he was withdrawing all UN Emergency troops from the Sinai Peninsula and the Gaza Strip, all at that time under Egyptian control. Israel waited with baited breath. Just a few days later, on May 23, another and much more sinister event occurred – Gamal Abdul Nasser closed the Straits of Tiran at Sharm el Sheik to Israeli shipping, thereby closing the passage to Israel's Red Sea port of Eilat in the Gulf of Aqaba. In a speech he made announcing this, he told his people that this may well lead to war with Israel, but that he was ready. This closure blocked Israel's sea route to the East. Israel had always said that such an act would be taken as a declaration of war and, once this happened, we all knew that war was inevitable. Israel had always been denied access to the Suez Canal, so that without the port of Eilat, shipping to and from the East had to go via the Mediterranean and Atlantic Oceans and around the Cape of Good Hope in South Africa. This was the vital strategic significance of Eilat. The country braced itself for what it now knew to be inevitable.

Only a matter of days later, there was a massive call up of reservists, myself included, and we were to remain in the army until about a month after what was to be called the Six Day War. We had a standing arrangement with my parents that whenever I was called to *miluim*, Jenny would go and stay with them, where she would receive lots of love and attention in my absence. Jenny is an incredibly serene person and in many ways the supreme optimist, and she tells me that she never believed that anything would happen to me. She was badly rattled by the anti-Israeli hate propaganda that was blaring over the radio from the neighboring Arab countries at that time, broadcast both in English and in Hebrew. Jenny's attitude and show of calm, plus the remarkable calm of my parents, made going off on this emergency call up much easier than it could have been. After all, this was not a regular call up for *miluim* – this was an *emergency* call up, and that was much more serious. However, later Jenny confessed that the morning I had to report, she dropped me off and went home and cried and cried.

Tension was high among the mobilized soldiers, but perhaps even higher among the civilian population because they had better access to the hideous and terrifying anti-Israel rhetoric that was pouring out of Jordanian, Syrian and Egyptian radio. We were not always near a radio, and so to a certain extent were protected from this vitriol.

If tension was high, then so was morale, too, although some of the troops were tense, and this was reflected in some soldiers' behavior when guarding. In a parallel company to mine, for example, a tragic event occurred: a reserve soldier just like me was on guard duty in the middle of the night, when he heard a noise behind him. It was one of the men in his platoon grunting in his sleep as he turned over in his sleeping bag. The guard aimed his Uzi sub-machine gun, and fired a burst in the direction of the grunts. The soldier was killed instantly – by a friend from his own platoon.

During those weeks that preceded the outbreak of the war, I got to know Dudu, my company commander, a major. Dudu was very different from most officers I encountered in *Tzahal*, and from the first day I met him while doing *miluim* about a year before the Six Day War, I realized that this man was a gem. He was an excellent commander, and could be as firm and as tough as the next man. However, on other occasions, he would show a very gentle, human side to his personality without this in any way undermining his status or authority with the soldiers under his command. It is therefore not surprising that he features in a number of my stories. He was a very competent but low-key, humane individual, who embodied all the positive aspects that I always see as distinguishing *Tzahal* and its commanders from most other armies. Dudu was thirty-five years old in 1967, but to me, aged twenty-three, he seemed old. He was not a large man, and certainly did not cut the image of the macho fighter that he actually was. He was soft-spoken, seldom raised his voice, and smoked incessantly. He was one of those rare and remarkable individuals who derive authority not from any external trait, but from their innate strength of character. Dudu managed to instill in me and in most of the rest of the company a sense of calm and confidence that '*hakol yihyeh beseder*' (Everything will be okay).

Not long after Dudu took over the command of our company, the rumor spread that he had been awarded a citation for bravery (*tzalash*) several years earlier. The Israeli army, to its credit, does not award medals, and since there is no visible symbol of an award there's no way of knowing about a *tzalash* unless one was present, or is told. The uniform of one of Dudu's men had, so the rumor went, caught fire after the man foolishly tried to refill a burning kerosene lamp. The lamp burst into flames and then exploded. Dudu rushed up to this man, who was by now a flaming torch, knocked him down and rolled on top of him to put out the fire. The soldier was very badly burned, but survived. Dudu never said a word about this feat of bravery, but I verified it when I met him in Jerusalem in 2002. He was most intrigued that we, his men, had somehow heard the story, because it was not in our unit and none of us had been present.

We were in the army from the day of the huge reserve call up, and were based in Jerusalem in an improvised camp in a public park in the southern suburbs of the city. Our families were allowed to visit us, and on Friday nights they were allowed to spend the evening with us. Dudu would give little speeches of encouragement to us on these Friday nights, and the theme was always the same: We are doing what we are doing solely to protect our homes and our loved ones. The speeches, like everything about Dudu, were always low-key, but at the same time extremely encouraging, positive, and sincere, and they meant a great deal to us.

Little did we know as we listened to his speeches that, within a fortnight, we were to be thrown into the heart of a critical battle in Jerusalem, a battle that was part of one of the most remarkable wars ever fought and that was to change the face and destiny of Israel forever. And I fought that war with Dudu's words resounding in my ears, especially as I knew that the distance from where I fought on the first day of the war to my home was no more than two miles.

About a week or less before the war began, we were moved to the area, maybe 10 miles outside Jerusalem, called the 'Jerusalem Corridor.' It lies very close to the Jordanian border, and is painfully vulnerable to attack. We set up camp there, and worked all day digging defensive trenches for the agricultural settlements in the area. Although the powers that be knew full well that war was inevitable and imminent we, or at least I, did not realize it or want to believe it. I think many of the other soldiers felt the same, because they behaved no differently from the way they behaved in any stint in *miluim*, often shirking or doing as little as possible. One guy, Moshe, a chronic shirker, kept telling us that he had cancer and that it was jumping around in his body. "Here it is in my arm. Wait a minute, it's moved to my chest," he would tell us, and we just laughed at him.

On the morning of June 5 we were wakened very early and told to pack up our equipment and to eat breakfast quickly, as we were being moved again – this time back into Jerusalem. As a lowly soldier not privy to what was being planned, I had no idea what awaited us, and simply assumed that it was yet another bureaucratic or logistical move, the logic of which escaped me. We grumpily loaded all our equipment and ourselves onto chartered buses and set off for Jerusalem. As we were beginning the final ascent to the city, Yossie, my platoon commander, stood up and shouted for us to keep quiet. "The war has begun," he shouted, "and if you listen you will hear the sounds of the artillery explosions in the area. The Jordanians are shelling Jerusalem and we are on our way into battle!"

The bus went deathly silent. Each of us began to think about what we had just been told, and to try to fathom its meaning.

The buses took us to Bak'a – a lovely old suburb in the southern part of Jewish Jerusalem. At a certain point, on some insignificant suburban street, the buses stopped and again Yossie stood up and shouted: "I want everybody to get off the bus, and to line up in threes so that I can check your equipment before we go into battle." We were just near the old Camp Allenby. This had served as a major British camp for the duration of the British Mandate in Palestine, and was in use at that time, I believe, by the Israeli police.

As we climbed off the bus, I realized that I had our transistor radio in my shirt pocket. It was one of those little radios, about the size of a cigarette box, which is worth very little today, but was quite a luxury in the Israel of those days. How could I go to war with this radio in my pocket? What would happen if we had to dive onto the ground or crawl? The radio might get damaged. You can see just how logical and sensible *I* was being at that moment. And then I had a brain wave: I rushed up to the door of one of the little houses in that Bak'a street and knocked. A woman opened it. There I stood, in full combat outfit, including helmet, hand grenades, stretcher – the works.

"I wonder if you could do me a favor? We are on our way into battle and I am worried about my radio getting broken. Would you look after it for me, please, and I will come and collect it after the war?"

Of course the woman agreed, and I rushed back to rejoin my platoon.

I thought a lot about that radio during the next month, and when I was discharged a few weeks after the end of the war, Jenny and I went to Bak'a to reclaim it. I did not know the name or number of the street, but after a couple of inquiries I found the building and rang the bell. I was clean-shaven, in neat civilian clothes and sandals. The same woman came to the door:

"Do you remember that a soldier came and asked you to look after his transistor radio for him on the first morning of the war?"

"Of course I remember", she replied.

"Well, I am that soldier and I have come to ask for my radio back, please."

The woman's eyes filled with tears. "We have been praying for you ever since you brought us the radio, and hoping that you would come back to claim it. *Baruch Haba* (Blessed be you in your coming.) But I am afraid we used up the batteries." We embraced, she gave me the radio, and I never saw her again, nor did we even learn each others' names.

We set off, on foot, from Bak'a and made our way eastwards towards the Jordanian border, which cut Jerusalem in two according to the Armistice agreement of 1949. We were walking towards the United Nations Headquarters for the Middle East, a building which had previously been the official residence of the British High Commissioner in Mandatory Palestine. In fact, the building to this day is known in Hebrew as *Armon Hanatziv* – the Commissioner's Palace, or Government House.

The U.N. Headquarters is an imposing building, set on its own two to three acres of grounds, and it was fenced off and designated as 'no-man's-land' – neither Israeli nor Jordanian territory. This United Nations compound, lying due south of the Old City of Jerusalem, was the nerve center and administrative headquarters of all UN operations in the Middle East. At this spot the Israel/Jordan border ran from north to south, with Israel extending to the west of the fenced area and Jordan extending to the east of it. What made this such a strategic position was that this circle of land perches on the brow of a hill, with the ground sloping downwards to the west into the western suburbs of Israeli Jerusalem, and downwards to the east into the Arab villages on the southern outskirts of Jordanian Jerusalem. This made it strategically very important and the Jordanians, knowing this, and knowing that there were no U.N. combat troops there but only non-combatant officials, overran the compound immediately the war began and ordered the U.N. personnel out. Many did leave, but a few opted instead to remain, huddling for shelter in the basement. The Old City of Jerusalem lies within easy shelling distance, separated only by the Kidron valley – as the crow flies no distance at all – so once installed in the U.N. compound, the Jordanian army began shelling the southern suburbs of Jerusalem – Bak'a, Talpiyot, the German Colony, Talbiyeh and Rechavia.

As we made our way eastwards, the noise of shelling became louder and louder. We mainly advanced in single file, and as the platoon medic I marched up front with Yossie, my platoon commander, and with Dudu, our company commander who happened to be advancing with our platoon. Suddenly, one of the sergeants came running up to Yossie and Dudu and said that Meir, one of the riflemen, was constantly falling behind. This was no time for playing games, and both officers were angry, as Meir had acquired an unenviable reputation for being a slacker. The sergeant reported, "He not only keeps falling behind, but he pretends not to understand me when I speak to him." After some discussion, focussing on the idea that what he really needed was a swift kick in the backside, Dudu sent me back to where Meir was to see what was going on. I, too, was in no mood for Meir's nonsense, and shouted to him to run to catch up with the platoon. He looked at me blankly, and gestured with his hands that he did not understand me and could not hear me. I tried again. Same thing. I ran back to Dudu and Yossie, and reported to them that I thought there was something wrong with him and that he should be evacuated.

"Nonsense," said Yossie. "He's just acting up again. I'm going back to push him to keep up."

I was not comfortable with this, but really had no basis other than my gut instinct to go by – our very brief medic's course, which focused exclusively on first aid in the field, in no way covered such cases. Moreover, I was a private, and the two men whose decision I was in effect challenging were a major and a lieutenant respectively. Thinking quickly, I said that I would do what they told me to, but that I thought that there was indeed a medical problem, and that Meir should be evacuated. Dudu immediately gave the order that Meir be evacuated to hospital. After the war, I inquired what had become of Meir, and learned that he had been admitted to a closed psychiatric ward of a city hospital suffering from shock brought on by the knowledge that he was going into battle. I later learned that this had resulted in a nine month period of hospitalization, during which he was stone deaf and uncommunicative, although his hearing was eventually restored. I did once bump into him in Jerusalem about a year after the war. He did not recognize me when I greeted him.

After about 20 minutes of rapid marching we reached an agricultural college next to the border. The college had an experimental farm, where they reared minks in cages in single-story corrugated iron shed-like buildings. We were told to lie down along the sides of these structures in which the minks were housed. Mortar shells began falling all around us – this was my first experience of being shelled, and of hearing the terrifying, high pitched whistle of the mortar shell as it descended, without knowing where exactly it was going to land. All you can do in such circumstances is put your head down and wait for it to land, and pray that it does not hit you. Such a shell does not need to land directly on you in order to kill or maim you – it's perfectly sufficient that it land near you, as it explodes on impact, spraying lethal fragments of shrapnel in all directions.

One of the officers explained to us that the Jordanians had taken control of the entire United Nations compound, and that they were planning on using this as a bridgehead into the southern suburbs of Israeli Jerusalem. We were going to have to root them out.

It was here at the agricultural college, for the first time in my life, for real and not as part of my medic's course, that I heard that terrible shout, "*Chovesh!*" – the call for help when someone is wounded. It was my friend Shimon, whose death I described at this book's beginning.

Apart from seeing the old grandfather of a family friend lying in his bed a few minutes after he had died when I was about fourteen, this was my first encounter with death. And, what is more, the one thing that they had not taught us in the medics' course was that when people in your unit are injured or killed and you are called to treat them, it is *friends* you are treating, not anonymous soldiers. That encounter with death was shattering, and in retrospect I don't know how I found the strength to pick myself up and carry on, but the human body is strong and resilient and can function almost apart from the mind, and somehow I just responded.

We waited at this agricultural college for some time, with mortar shells constantly exploding all around. I subsequently learned that, during this time, the Israeli artillery had been shelling the Jordanians in the compound. We then began to advance again in the direction of the U.N. Headquarters. Just near the entrance to the compound was a small wood of evergreen trees, many of which were on fire from exploding shells, and we were advancing between them. This made the scene positively surreal. As we advanced through the stone arch at the entrance to the compound, a soldier in front of me was hit by a bullet and fell dead at my feet.

After some fierce fighting we were finally able to force our way into the compound, and then fanned out to the south of the building. In due course the firing stopped, as the Jordanian soldiers had either been killed – many lay dead all around as we advanced – had retreated, or had surrendered.

At one point I noticed Asher, our battalion commander who had led the entire force attacking the U.N. Headquarters, shouting orders to officers, and waving only one of his arms as he did so. There was a thin trickle of blood running down his arm. I prepared a sterile bandage and rushed up to him, yelling "Just stay still for two minutes while I bandage your arm!"

"Leave me alone! Can't you see I'm very busy?" he yelled back belligerently.

But I persisted and ultimately he let me bandage his arm – a bullet had gone right through it, and I was able to identify the entry and exit holes quite easily. What I did not know, however, was that in fact the bullet had severed the nerves in his arm, and done critical damage. Asher must have known that something was seriously wrong with his arm, but he ignored it and continued to command, only reluctantly agreeing the next day to be finally evacuated to hospital. Several months later, Asher's name appeared in the newspaper as a recipient of one of the 55 citations by the commander-in-chief, Yitzchak Rabin. This was the highest of three levels of citations awarded after the Six Day War, with the other two levels being by divisional and brigade commanders. Learning that Asher was one of the recipients of the commander-in chief's awards brought home to us just how important that victory at the U.N. Headquarters had been in determining the outcome of the war on the Jordanian front. But we also learned that Asher had lost partial use of that arm, had to retire from commanding a combat unit, and ended up as a military advisor.

The details of what I experienced that day are as clear these 36 years later as they were then. Of course I was not aware of or privy to the bigger picture. For example, I know that other units from my battalion took part in the battle, but I do not know the details. What I do know is that by around 4.00 p.m. on that first day we had retaken the United Nations Headquarters and driven out the Jordanians, and the danger of a Jordanian invasion into the southern suburbs of Jerusalem had been averted.

During that traumatic first day, I attended to several wounded and dead soldiers, some from my unit, some from other units. By the end of that day's fighting my clothes, as well as my hands and arms, were completely drenched in blood – with no chance to wash. It was not that my clothes were spattered with blood like a painter's overall – they were soaked in blood, caked *all over* with blood, as if my pants and shirt had been dipped into a tub of red paint. In fact, I presented such a revolting sight to the other infantrymen that they somehow found a pair of pants and a shirt form me to change into.

We were positioned all around the building in the U.N. grounds, and were told to dig in – to dig foxholes for ourselves, those shallow graves that infantry soldiers lie in when the unit is not on the move, since it gives them some protection. As a medic, I was required to dig a double foxhole – one for me, and one for any wounded soldier I might have to look after. In June in Israel it is already very dry, and the ground is rock hard. The digging was not easy, especially as we dug with small World War Two folding trench shovels, on our knees, so as not to be too exposed to Jordanian positions across the valley.

Early that Monday morning Jenny was at work, and when the air raid sirens sounded in Jerusalem she and her co-workers went down to the underground shelving areas for shelter. When, later, the all clear sounded, she immediately drove back to my parents' apartment where she was staying, and together they all went down to the bomb shelter of their apartment building as soon as the next air raid alert was sounded. While there are public shelters in Jerusalem, the city's building code requires that in addition every building have a shelter constructed according to certain established specifications.

Meanwhile, a world away in South Africa, Steve and Ami waited anxiously for news from Israel. What we subsequently learned was that there had been a news blackout imposed by *Tzahal* for almost the entire day; the first news of the progress of the war reported on Israel Radio was of Jordan's occupation of the U.N. Headquarters, and of *Tzahal*'s subsequent capture of the compound and routing of the Jordanian army from there. Jenny and my parents, sitting in the air raid shelter, heard this good news, as did everyone in the country who was not mobilized, but little did she know that her husband had been in the thick of the battle – it was to be several days before I was able to make contact. As far as she knew, I was still in the 'Jerusalem Corridor' where we had spent the previous week.

Not only did we not listen to the radio, neither did we eat or drink on that first day, except for that very early breakfast we ate before returning to Jerusalem, and for the water we had in our canteens. Later that first night, I was sent with a group of soldiers back to where we had left our battalion's heavy equipment at Camp Allenby, and *en route* we stopped at the agricultural college through which we had advanced. We were by now ravenously hungry, as it was about 14 hours since we'd eaten. We asked them for some food, but all they had themselves were some dry crackers, which they willingly gave us, and which we just as gladly ate.

That same night I found a bow tie on an elastic, which presumably must have belonged to some U.N. official. It was lying on the ground near the U.N. building. The discovery amidst the chaos of war of this brightly patterned piece of haberdashery, an almost defiantly civilian article of dress so far removed from our world of the battlefield, struck me as comical in the extreme. Overwhelmed by the wild incongruity of it all, I went and attached it to the filthy uniform of one of our new officers, a lieutenant who was bringing up the heavy equipment. Called Yossie like our platoon commander, he and I had become quite friendly with each other over the period that we had been mobilized. He, too, appreciated the mad comedy of it all, and walked around all night proudly sporting the bow tie.

We spent that first night guarding, digging and sleeping as best we could in shifts. We slept in our foxholes, with nothing more than a shirt and pants on, and no blankets, and although it was early summer it was quite cold that night on the hill. Jerusalem being high up is cool in the evenings, and our hilltop was a fairly exposed one. I am sure that exhaustion and lack of food did not help.

Some time in the morning Yossie, the platoon commander, came by and informed us that we had to abandon our carefully dug foxholes and dig new ones about 15 meters away. The reason was that with daylight he had been able to discern that where we were dug in was visible across the valley in Jordan. As you can imagine, he was not popular, as the digging had been hard work. But an order is an order, and grumbling and complaining we began digging once again. By sunset that day, we were all blessing Yossie and his foresight and brilliance in moving us, as it saved many of our lives when the Jordanians opened fire from a tank directly across the valley.

Around lunch time some drinking water and some battle-ration crackers were brought to us. But I was still covered with dried blood. Despite the change of clothes, I had had no way of washing the blood off my arms and hands, and I was revolted at the prospect of handling the food and then putting it into my mouth. So I persuaded one of the people in my platoon to feed me.

Later on that day, the Yossie of bow tie fame came down to my foxhole to talk to me. I say 'down' because our battalion headquarters and *ta'agad* were inside the U.N. building, and we were dug in on the grounds that sloped downwards into Jordan. My particular foxhole faced roughly north-east.

Yossie was not a regular member of our battalion – indeed I'd never met him before he suddenly appeared a few days before the outbreak of the war. It turned out that he had been in the United States for an extended period doing a Ph.D., and had very recently returned to Israel. So recently, in fact, that *Tzahal* had not yet placed him in a unit, but when this state of emergency began, he volunteered and was seconded to our battalion. He was an extremely nice guy, and we struck up a friendship almost immediately. Not being a regular officer in the battalion, he was a 'floater' and carried out various tasks as they arose. I don't know exactly what he had been sent down the line for, but in any case I was very pleased that he stopped to visit me in my foxhole. It was still unsafe to stand around, as there remained substantial danger from Jordanian tanks and snipers, so we lay in my double foxhole. He told me that he had heard that the area of the Hebrew University, Givat Ram campus, had been shelled and had suffered some damage, but he knew no details. At the time this was very upsetting to me as that was exactly where Jenny worked, and my school was directly adjacent. (I subsequently learned that Jenny was safely in the shelter at my parents' apartment building and not at work at all, and that the kids in the schools were all rushed into shelters the moment the siren went off. As a result, no one was injured, although the school suffered a direct hit when an artillery shell crashed through its roof.) Yossie and I chatted for a while, and then he said he had some things to attend to while down on the line and he had better go.

My foxhole was deliberately set about 30 feet back from the rest of the platoon in case I had to treat someone right there. Yossie ran from my foxhole to that of one of the sergeants in our platoon, and lay down to talk to him. Not ten minutes later, we were suddenly shelled by a tank, and within moments that terrible scream, "*Chovesh!*" was coming from all directions, including Yossie's. I rushed across, and there lay Yossie, mortally wounded. I began to examine him but, within seconds, he gasped his last breath. He died in my arms. Close by lay a second soldier, also dead.

Israel is really a very small country, even today but certainly more so in 1967. One evening in the 1980's we went to a lecture given by Yael

Dayan in Toronto, and as we were filing into the hall we heard the people in front of us talking Hebrew. We chimed in, and it emerged that they were from Jerusalem. After the lecture we invited them home for coffee. As it turned out, we shared much in common – Roni is also an academic, we had all been at the Hebrew University around the same time, and Puah even remembered Jenny's and my blossoming romance in the English Department. In due course, in inevitable Israeli fashion, conversation turned to the army and where we had served. When I said "Jerusalem," Roni asked,

"Jerusalem? Did you know my first cousin, Yossie L.?" I felt a cold shiver run down my spine.

"Yossie died in my arms," I told them, a lump forming in my throat.

As a *chovesh* with minimal training, I was not allowed to declare a soldier dead, even when he obviously was. Army regulations called for us to continue to treat these men as 'the most seriously wounded.' That regulation would have been all very fine and large, except that there were some twelve soldiers wounded in that sudden shelling, some very seriously, including one bleeding profusely from a huge gash in his back, a piece of shrapnel having hit him as he lay on his stomach in his foxhole. Their cries for help were almost unendurable. I was alone with the soldiers of my platoon – no other medic in sight, let alone a doctor, and the shelling around us was continuing unabated. I have no idea where our company medic was at that moment. I had to make a split-second decision: Do I follow army regulations and continue to attend to Yossie and the other dead soldier, or do I abandon them and attend to the others? I could not, in all conscience, let the infantryman with the back wound simply lie there and bleed to death, fully conscious, when stopping the bleeding was something we had been taught and which was relatively simple to perform. In other words, then, not so very hard a decision to make after all.

Someone ran to me and told me that there was an underground air raid shelter not far away in the grounds. "Pick up the wounded and bring them into the shelter," I shouted. The shelter was built with a narrow flight of stairs down to it, and it was a very small room, quite dark, about 15 feet long and about nine or ten feet wide. There were stone benches built along the length of the shelter on both sides, leaving an open floor width of about four feet. We began bringing the wounded in, and it was pandemonium. There were soldiers shouting, some moaning and several crying hysterically. One man, an immigrant from Yemen, was uncontrollable – it was his friend who, along with Yossie, had taken a direct hit and been killed outright. These two men had come to Israel without their families in 'Operation Magic Carpet,' when the brand-new State of Israel had airlifted over ninety-five percent of the Yemenite Jewish community from Aden to Israel and safety in May, 1949. Having come without their families, they had become like brothers to each other, lived close to each other in Ein Karem – a suburb of Jerusalem – and made an honorable living as partners in a house-painting business. He knew that his friend, whom he referred to as his 'brother,' was dead.

Everyone was shouting instructions to everyone else as they tried to get the wounded down the narrow steps and into the shelter. Some of the wounded were crying, one man was screaming that he was blind, and I was trying to attend to them as best I could. To make things even more difficult, I had had them place Benny, the man with the gash in his back, on the floor between the two rows of fixed stone benches which were already filled with other, equally seriously wounded, soldiers. Conditions were so cramped that some of the wounded had to lift up their feet so that Benny could find space to lie on the floor. It all meant that there was barely room enough room for me to put my own foot down without standing on Benny. Suddenly there was a very loud shout from the steps:

"*Sheket!*" ("Be quiet!") It was Dudu. He had come down to the line to see what was going on after the shelling.

"Listen up," he ordered. "From this moment, every word that comes out of David's mouth is a direct order from me."

Everyone quieted down immediately. Suddenly, and thanks to Dudu, I found myself with the authority to control the situation.

I began attending to the gash in Benny's back. I had been trained that the way to stop the bleeding, unless it was arterial, was to put a pressure bandage on the wound and to bind it very tightly. I grabbed a magazine of bullets from one of the soldiers and used that to apply pressure on the wound, and then had to tie a bandage around his whole torso so that the magazine was hard against the wound. Benny was in his thirties, and somewhat overweight, but he was also very brave. I explained to him that I was going to tie this bandage around him, and that it would hurt, and would pinch the skin as I had to tie it very tightly. "Not a problem," he said, "do it." I tied the bandage around his ample body, and then began to pull it tighter and tighter. In fact, to get it tight enough, I actually put my boot against his side to give me leverage. I know that this pinched the skin under his arm terribly, as we had practiced this with each other in training, but there we had been taught to apply carefully a bandage or something to prevent pinching the skin. I neither had the time nor the bandage to do that, and Benny understood. He never said a word or let out a sound, except to thank me when it was safely tied. Benny was then evacuated, and was successfully operated on. I saw him a few months later, and he was doing fine. We remained in contact for several years, and he would tell me that the only ill-effect he was left with was a twinge now and then in the area of the wound when the weather changed.

Slowly, I began treating all the wounded in order of severity according to the triage training we had been given. Although things gradually began to calm down, it was still not that easy: I was still alone, and what is more, I had totally run out of sterile dressings of *any* size, and was dressing open wounds with unsterile bandages and even, towards the end when these, too, ran out, with one of the soldiers' shirts which I cut up. We finally evacuated them all up the hill to our *ta'agad*. I say 'we,' but of course I couldn't be part of the evacuation process as the *chovesh* has to remain on the line.

That mass injury on the second day of the Six Day War was the most terrible day of my life. The training I had received was minimal, and there I was, alone, having to make these life and death decisions. I had nightmares for months afterwards, and in my nightmare I was being court-martialed for contravening army regulations and thereby causing death – for abandoning the two dead guys and attending to the others. Paradoxically, what actually happened was that Dudu recommended me for a citation for my actions that fateful day. I never did receive one – few were awarded out of a pool of some two and a half thousand nominees, but to have been nominated was itself a great honor, and I feel to this day like an actor who has been nominated for an Oscar. What is interesting is that the next day, after the fighting at the U.N. Headquarters had stopped, I cracked. I began to cry hysterically, and had to be taken to the *ta'agad* and given some sedation. I was kept under the watchful eye of the doctor in the *ta'agad* for several hours, after which I was fine and was able to return to my platoon and to duty.

Perhaps you'll recall that when I was talking about being sent on a medic's course, I explained that being a medic was low-status and that we were treated almost with disdain. Well, by the end of the war's first day that had all changed, and I found myself treated with much love, affection, and respect by the rest of the platoon, evidenced for example by the one man's willingness to feed me those crackers when my unwashed hands were coated with blooded. There were many sincere expressions of appreciation from the platoon for my work as a chovesh, and while these may have embarrassed me, at the same time I was deeply touched.

We remained dug in around the U.N. Headquarters until June 7. Thank goodness there was no more shelling directly at us, but we were acutely aware that there was still heavy fighting in several areas around the Old City. We also knew that the Jordanians were holding firm within the Old City itself. At one point, there was a rumor that the Jordanians were mounting a counterattack on the U.N. compound from the valley separating the compound from the Old City to the north. Our officers called for volunteers to crawl from where we were dug in to look over the brow of the hill to observe any Jordanian troop movement in our direction. This was a daunting prospect, as these men could have found themselves suddenly face to face with any advancing counterattacking force. A friend of mine, Barry, originally from Cape Town, was one of those who volunteered. We all held our breath as they crawled northward towards the brow of the hill. After what seemed like an eternity, they returned safely and reported that there were absolutely no troops advancing in our direction, and that it had all been a false alarm.

While I was recovering in the *ta'agad*, I went for a walk around the splendid U.N. building. Looking into one room, I saw that it was an office and that there was a sheet of paper in the typewriter. I went in and had a look. I could hardly believe it. It was an official report that had been typed, on U.N. letterhead, stating that war had broken out in the Middle East. I guess it was something that was then going to be sent by telex or radio. I decided that it would make a very nice souvenir, and I folded it up and put it into my pocket. Unfortunately, the following day, in a personal and private moment, doing what has to be done, I realized I had no toilet paper or, indeed, any paper at all. And then I remembered the U.N. document, and forthwith put it to good use. A sad fate for a historic document, and I could kick myself today.

Being on a hill across the valley from the Old City gave us a spectacular view of what was going on. At that point, the Old City had not yet been captured. That first night, we watched as the roof of the Dormition Abbey burned on Mount Zion after a mortar shell had come crashing through it. It was a bit like watching a grimly realistic *son et lumière*. Then, on the morning of June 7, we heard announcements in Arabic coming over loudspeakers being broadcast from Israeli army jeeps. Several of the men in my platoon knew Arabic and they translated:

"Jordanian soldiers in the Old City! We call on you to surrender. You are surrounded. The United Nations Headquarters (to the south) is in Israeli hands; the Mount of Olives (to the east) is in Israeli hands, Mount Scopus and Augusta Victoria (to the north-east) are in Israeli hands; all the high points surrounding the Old City are in Israeli hands."

And of course, as they and we all knew full well, directly to the west of the Old City was Israel itself. These broadcasts went on for some time, and it was eerie listening to them coming clear across the valley in an otherwise silent city where people were not venturing out on either side yet.

But the Jordanians did not surrender. This left Israel with two choices if it wished to capture the Old City: to bombard it from outside with artillery and even from the air, which would take the smallest toll in Israeli lives, or to send in infantry to do the job, street-by-street. It is a tribute to *Tzahal*, the unique army that it is, that they decided on the latter approach in order not to damage the large number of holy shrines in the Old City – shrines sacred to all three of the major monotheistic religions in the world: the El Aksa and Dome of the Rock mosques on the Temple Mount, the Church of the Holy Sepulchre and the Via Dolorosa – the street Christ walked to his crucifixion – and the Western Wall of the Second Temple, so holy to Jews – to name only the most important ones. This approach, dedicated to preserving the sites holy to *all* the religions represented, was very different from that of the Jordanians who had ruled East Jerusalem since the 1949 Armistice agreement. They desecrated most of the Jewish holy sites, including virtually the entire Jewish Quarter of the Old City and the Jewish cemetery on the slopes of the Mount of Olives. Surprisingly, the Western Wall remained intact.

And so it was that Motta Gur's paratroopers entered the Old City on foot, fighting a street-by-street battle until the valiant Jordanian army had been overcome and the Old City liberated. It was at this point that *Tzahal*'s Chief Rabbi, Shlomo Goren, accompanied by Defense Minister Moshe Dayan, came to the Western Wall, and there was the historic blowing of the shofar (ram's horn) to mark the liberation. Despite our vantage point, we were not aware of what was going on because the paratroopers entered through a gate to the east of the Old City, which we could not see from where we were. Neither is it possible to see into the Old City from outside because of the walls. So we, like the rest of the nation, ultimately learned the news from the radio.

On June 7, we moved south from the U.N. Headquarters to Bethlehem. Having lived with the 1949 Armistice borders ever since I came to Israel, I had no idea how close Bethlehem was to Jerusalem. Our clumsy and plodding convoy crept slowly southwards to Bethlehem that day, using the old British Mandatory road that entered East Jerusalem just east of the U.N. Headquarters, and encountering all sorts of difficulties along the way, as the road had been mined and booby-trapped in several places by the retreating Jordanian army. One of our vehicles detonated a mine, killing one soldier and injuring two. The trip took several hours, and we only reached Bethlehem after dark, to be greeted by a sea of white flags of surrender, and not a Jordanian soldier, nor indeed any other person, in sight. A deathly silent city. We made our way to Manger Square, opposite the Church of the Nativity, which is built on the spot where it is believed Christ was born, and went into the police station on the square. We could hear loud and frantic shouting – the Jordanian police had run away, leaving the people they were holding in custody locked in their cells without food or water. I don't know how long they had been left alone like that, but this was yet another surrealistic component of that day. It was in the police station that I found a discarded Jordanian army red and white *keffiyah* (head scarf), which I have kept to this day.

We slept the night in the police station, and the following morning were told to shave and to polish our boots for a battalion parade – our first opportunity to wash and shave for four days. It is amazing how important being clean shaven for the first time in four days and having polished boots was – our clothes were filthy, we hadn't showered or washed since before the start of the war, and yet this made us feel human again, somehow contriving to restore our self-esteem.

We lined up in a hollow square formation in Manger Square, and were addressed by the battalion commander who had replaced the injured Asher. "Yesterday, the Old City of Jerusalem and the Western Wall were liberated, and last night a cease-fire came into effect with Jordan." Without another word or command, we all spontaneously came to attention and, with tears in our eyes, sang *Hatikva*, the Israeli national anthem.

There were many strange moments while we were stationed in Bethlehem. That morning, we were allowed to walk around Manger Square in groups for safety's sake, and to visit the Church of the Nativity and the surrounding tourist shops. We went into the Church of the Nativity, and saw a man sweeping up debris. On looking up, we understood – it was debris from a shell that had crashed through the roof of the church.

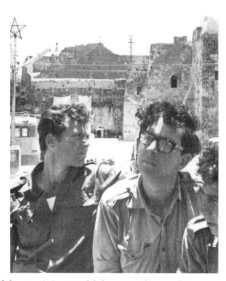

At the Church of the Nativity, Bethlehem, with my platoon commander, Yossie; June, 1967

A day or so later, the frightened citizens of Bethlehem began to emerge from their houses, not at all sure what was going to happen. I have always been an idealist and a dreamer, and I believe to this day that in spite of the hardening of attitudes that sadly has taken place over the years, the Israeli army has always functioned on a higher moral plane than most armies. So I am proud to record that *absolutely nothing* happened to these people. They were not harassed, there was no rape or violence, and there was no looting. In fact, when the tourist shops with all their little olive wood camels and other trinkets began to open, we bought small gifts to take home to our families. The shopkeepers were dumbfounded. They had expected us to refuse to pay. My purchase from one of those stores was of a beautiful lampshade made of Hebron glass beads; it still graces our living room in Toronto, giving off a special light due to the exquisite blue of the glass beads. Over the subsequent years George, the owner of that gift store, and I became friends, and Jenny and I would drive out to Bethlehem to buy gifts from him whenever something was needed.

After that first night in the police station we were moved to a school, where we slept like sardines in a can, one next to the other on the floor in a classroom. The school had a flat roof on which we did guard duty.

On one of the nights, I was wakened for my stint of guarding in the middle of the night, and dragged myself onto the roof. When I was relieved and came back to the classroom, I noticed Moshe, the guy who told us about his 'traveling cancer,' sitting up smoking a cigarette. Everyone else was sound asleep. Moshe was always a bit weird, so I thought nothing of it and went straight to sleep. I was wakened from a deep sleep by a terribly loud explosion in our room. There was no electricity, it was pitch dark, and pandemonium broke out. We thought a hand grenade had been tossed in through the window. Suddenly I heard what by then had become an all too familiar cry:

"*Chovesh!*"

It was Moshe – this had not been an attack from outside, neither had it been a hand grenade – it just sounded like that to us, fast asleep in this hollow room. Moshe had shot himself with his own rifle. Whether he intended to kill himself, or whether this was a cry for help, we will never know, but he shot himself in the stomach, injuring his internal organs terribly. We dressed his gaping stomach wound, and he was rushed to hospital. I never saw him again, and the last I ever heard of him was that he was living permanently in a closed psychiatric ward in a hospital.

The evening after we had reached Bethlehem, on June 8, around supper time, I approached my company commander, Dudu.

"You know, Dudu, our families have no idea where we are or whether we are safe or not. Isn't it possible for some of us to nip into Jerusalem and go around to people's homes and at least inform the families that we are okay? After all, things here are quiet."

In those days, very few people had telephones, hence my proposal that we should go house to house. To my delight, Dudu agreed. Of course I wasn't really all that surprised, as in addition to being an exemplary soldier he is a most compassionate and humane man.

"Go and find four more people who have cars who are willing to drive around from address to address informing the families. I'll get the company clerk to prepare lists of names and addresses. Mind you, he has to be very careful to eliminate the names of all the dead and the wounded – the last thing we need is for one of you to go to one of those houses. I'll arrange transportation to Jerusalem for you after supper."

I had no difficulty finding four others who owned cars and were willing to participate, as the prospect of going back to Jerusalem, even if only for a few hours, and seeing our families and telling them personally that we were well, was intoxicating.

A couple of hours later, the five of us set out in a company command car, each equipped with a list of some 20 names – a lot to cope with in blacked-out Jerusalem which, at the best of times, is not a city renowned for clear signage of street names and numbers. After all, this was only the fourth day of the war. People were no longer still in shelters, but the blackout was strictly enforced, which not only meant that it was pitch dark, but that the headlights of the command car had been painted over so that they provided only the faintest glow of light.

Just as we were about to leave for Jerusalem, one of the men in my platoon came up to me and said,

"I need you to do me a favor. I 'found' this radio in the U.N. building, and want you to take it home to your house tonight. I'll collect it after the war. You see, I'm worried that once they start to give us regular leave, they'll begin to check for things like this. I've stuffed the radio into a clean sandbag under the seat of the command car."

In the event, when we arrived and I was dropped off to pick up my car, I was so excited at the prospect of seeing Jenny and my parents that I totally forgot the radio, and it went sailing back to Bethlehem in the command car. I don't think it ever made it to Jerusalem. I guess this is justice of a kind, although one not calculated to make me popular.

We drove to Jerusalem along a different road, slightly to the west of the one we'd taken to get from the U.N. Headquarters to Jerusalem. This is actually the main road that is used today, which goes almost due north from Bethlehem, past Mar Elias Monastery and into the West Jerusalem suburb of Talpiyot. Remember that this was the first time I had ever been to Bethlehem, and all I knew of it was what you could glimpse from the lookout point at Kibbutz Ramat Rachel, where we always took our overseas visitors. After all, for me, Bethlehem had always been in Jordan – an enemy country.

We drove in the pitch dark with our dimmed, painted-over headlights. Only two days prior to this we had advanced to Bethlehem along a much longer and more winding road, a journey that had taken our convoy many hours; now, despite the dark, we were traveling fast and, encountering no traffic whatsoever, within fifteen minutes found ourselves back in Jerusalem. What a welcome sight!

We were dropped at our homes, where we were to pick up our cars and go around telling the news to the families on our lists, meeting at a central point some four hours later – well past midnight.

The command car dropped me at the entrance to my parents' building near the military cemetery at Mount Herzl, where I knew Jenny was staying. My heart was pounding as, filthy dirty but tingling with excited anticipation, I trudged up the four flights of stairs. They had no idea I was coming. This was not a time for visitors, and the city streets were still deserted. I rang the doorbell and quickly called through the door that it was me. What a reception I received! We hugged and hugged, and I was as happy to know that they were all well as they were to see me. Jerusalem had been bombarded, and they had spent a couple of days in the shelters; like me, they had just come through a terrifying few days. I quickly explained why I was there, and that I was taking Jenny with me to visit the families on my list. But not before my mother served me a wonderful meal – I have no idea how she happened to have food virtually ready, but I was not in the least surprised as this was the norm with her. As students, we would regularly arrive home from university for supper accompanied by one, two, or sometimes more friends – always unannounced, yet somehow neither my hard working and devoted mother nor my easygoing father were one bit fazed. They were truly remarkable – here they were, living in a tiny government-subsidized apartment, on the fourth floor of a building with no elevator, in a country which was, at that time, substantially less developed than the South Africa they had left behind. And then, to crown everything, their younger son had gone off to fight in the front line in a war.

That evening, the moment he had a chance, my father told me the following story. My mother was famous in the family for being fanatical about cleanliness – witness her rush to take a bath when they arrived in Netanya from South Africa. We always used to pull her leg, because never a day went by without her washing her glasses with soap and water. Well, after they had all been confined to the air raid shelter for two days, the all clear signal was given and they were allowed to go back to their apartment. Knowing how frantic my mother would be to have a bath, my father told her to go ahead and have the first bath.

"It's quite alright, dear," she said, "You or Jenny can go first."

Jenny and my father were dumbfounded. They stared at each other in frank disbelief.

"There's something strange going on," my father said. "Please explain."

And very sheepishly my mother did so.

"Well, you see, when they said I could rush upstairs to get some food to take down to the shelter, I didn't tell you, but I quickly had a bath."

So my mother had taken a bath on the top floor of a building, in the middle of Jerusalem, while it was being shelled.

I ate quickly, and then Jenny and I set out in our car to do our rounds. This gave us a few precious hours together.

And so began our strange mission. But we had no idea quite how strange it was going to be.

We stumbled and fumbled our way in the dark, deserted streets, looking for the different addresses on my list, and it was not easy. Many of the people in my company, like me, were new immigrants, living in large government-sponsored housing complexes like ours. These were called *shikunim* – Israel's public housing – four story buildings (so no elevator was required), but as many as eight entrances, all identical, and the numbering poorly marked. It was starting to become late to be knocking on strangers' doors, especially in a black-out situation, and people were in any case still highly nervous, especially those who lived close to where the border had been. In addition, many people thought a visit from a stranger in army uniform meant the delivery of bad news, and it took some persuasion to get some of the families to open their doors at all. On several occasions, I had to shout my explanation as to why I was there through the door before they would open it. Once they understood who I was and why I was there, I was welcomed with open arms and hugs, and they all tried to get me to stay for something to eat and drink. Generally, Jenny stayed in the car when I went up to the different apartments, as we had a long list to get through and time was short.

One of the people on my list was Habib. He and I had been friends for several years in *miluim*. He was from North Africa, and we had a standing joke that our friendship was so important because "we Africans must stick together."

Habib was one of the men who lived in a *shikun* right on the old border near Ammunition Hill, which was the site of one of the most intensive battles of the war. After no small amount of difficulty I found the right building, the right entrance and the right apartment door, and knocked.

"Who is it?" someone asked suspiciously.

"It's David, a friend of Habib's from the army, and I've come to give you regards from Habib."

Silence. And then,

"Habib's dead," they shouted. "Go away."

"Habib's *not* dead," I replied in shock.

"Habib's dead. Go away!"

"What do you mean Habib's dead?" I asked, still through the door. "He's absolutely fine. We're in the same platoon. Trust me."

This went backwards and forwards for some time until they finally agreed to open the door.

The family had begun sitting *shiva* and were, as is the custom, sitting on the floor. *Shiva* is the traditional Jewish seven days of mourning that begins after someone's burial.

"We know that Habib is dead because someone we know saw his dead body being carried into Hadassah Hospital on the first day of the war."

"You're wrong," I half shouted.

"Prove it," they challenged me.

I was stumped. But then I had a brainwave.

"Habib has two children, right?"

"Right."

"And the older one is a little boy of about six, and the younger one is a little girl of about three. Right?"

"Right."

"And the boy dressed up as a cowboy for the Purim carnival at his school this year, and the little girl dressed up as a bunny rabbit. Right?"

"How on earth do you know?" they asked incredulously.

"Because Habib and I are good friends and just this evening, while we were eating our supper, he happened to show me the pictures of the children in his wallet."

At that point, Habib's mother fainted and slumped to the floor, and his father and his wife and sisters began crying and shouting and hugging me.

"You brought our Habib back to life for us," they shouted. 'We want to buy you the biggest present we can think of!"

I finally told them that they need not buy me anything, but every time I saw Habib after that he would insist that his family wanted to buy me a present.

I literally staggered out of that apartment, moved and shaken by this unique experience, and barely able to tell Jenny what had happened. We then continued on our rounds, and were welcomed so joyfully by each and every family we visited. Sadly, no one was able to make a similar visit to the families of Shimon, Yossie and the others who had died in the fighting.

In the early hours of the morning, Jenny dropped me back at our meeting point to return to Bethlehem, and she returned to my parents' apartment. I've often wondered what the three of them said to each other when she got home.

Israelis are remarkable people, and they seem to produce the best songs in times of trouble. And the Six Day War gave birth to some superb songs, which were played on the radio over and over again, and were sung by all of us. Some were poignant, like the song which is a letter from a *miluimnik* to his daughter telling her to be a good girl and to look after Mummy while he is away fighting in the war, and some were very funny like " Nasser is waiting for Rabin, Ay, yay, yay...," which mocks Nasser and the Egyptian army and somewhat crudely describes how Yitzchak Rabin is going to stick it to him .

There is a strong consciousness in *Tzahal* that the majority of the soldiers are civilians – reservists – and every effort is made to make their time in the army as pleasant as possible. As soon as circumstances allowed, we began being treated to performances by different entertainers and entertainment groups, the highlight of which, in all my time in *miluim*, was a performance by Naomi Shemer herself, singing her own songs. This took place in front of a packed audience of soldiers in a Bethlehem cinema. I love Naomi Shemer's songs, and I have always been a great fan of hers. Her songs are not only delightful, but they are always intensely poignant, perfectly capturing the mood and spirit of the country at that moment. For example, she wrote *The Two of Us Are from the Same Village* (*Anachnu mi'oto hakfar*) about two boys who grew up in the same village, went to school together, went into the army together and how one was killed and was brought back to the village to be buried. That song is played every Remembrance Day, and I have never heard it without it bringing tears to my eyes.

We all waited expectantly to hear Naomi Shemer sing her much loved *Jerusalem of Gold*, not knowing what was coming. After singing a number of other songs, Naomi Shemer announced that when the Old City and the Western Wall were liberated, she had written two new verses for *Jerusalem of Gold*. Her song of yearning for those places and not being able to go there now climaxed with the wondrous news that we could once again visit them, and go down through East Jerusalem via Jericho to the Dead Sea. She told us that she was dedicating these new verses to the soldiers who had fought for, but did not live to see, the liberation of Jerusalem. She proceeded to sing the song to a spellbound audience, complete with the two new verses, and as it finished we burst into wild applause and a standing ovation for many minutes, many of us with tears streaming down our faces. I will never forget that moment. And, miraculously, that performance was recorded live, and the record was sold and is still played on the radio on many occasions. The following is an English translation of the words of the added verses:

The wells are filled again with water,
The square with joyous crowd,
On the Temple Mount within the City,
The shofar rings out loud.

Chorus

Oh, Jerusalem of gold, and of light and of bronze,
I am the lute for all your songs.

Within the caverns in the mountains
A thousand suns will glow,
We'll take the Dead Sea road together
That runs through Jericho.

Chorus

    There is nothing that a *miluim* soldier wants and craves more than leave. And this longing is all the more intense when it is not a regular stint of *miluim*, but rather a war. The only leave I had had since the pre-war call up – if you can call it leave – was the three hour break while we were still encamped in Jerusalem, to enable us to go home and shower. Eventually, after a couple of weeks, the army began giving us leave, one at a time, for 24 hours. Only one person per platoon was allowed to be away at a time. The person going on leave was taken from the restricted military zone where we were into Jerusalem by army vehicle, and was then brought back the following day. The next person to go on leave would travel to Jerusalem in the vehicle picking up the returning soldier, but only when the previous soldier had reported at the meeting point was the next one allowed to set out for home.

    The riflemen drew lots to determine the order. It was particularly complicated for us *chovshim* to get leave, as every platoon only had one *chovesh* and there always had to be one on duty, so a medic had to be loaned to the platoon in question from the *ta'agad* until the platoon's own medic returned.

After what seemed like an age, my turn came. We were dropped in town around 9.00 in the morning. I knew that there was no point in going home, as Jenny would be at work at the Jewish National and University Library on the Givat Ram University campus. So I went straight to her office and met her there, and we spent some time together. I then called my parents at their respective offices, after which I wanted to go and greet my friends at the Hebrew University High School where I taught English, and conveniently enough this was right next door to the Givat Ram campus.

I walked into the entrance lobby of the school, filthy dirty, in full battle gear, helmet in my hand, and was given a warm welcome by staff and students alike. I was amazed to see the huge gaping hole in the roof of the school auditorium from a Jordanian shell that had torn through it during the first days of the war when, thank goodness, the students and staff were safely in the air raid shelters.

As I was standing chatting excitedly with some of the teachers, Mr. Bargur, the very serious middle-aged school secretary, came over and asked to speak to me. I was puzzled. He was not the friendliest of people on the staff, so much so that I never knew his first name, which was highly unusual for Israel – often one did not know a last name, but I can't think of another situation in which I *only* knew the last name.

"You haven't handed in your end of year grades for the twelfth graders," he reprimanded me. (The system in the twelfth grade was that the class teacher submitted a grade for each student, which was factored in with the student's grade in the state matriculation examination ("bagrut") to determine their school leaving final grade.)

"I'm terribly sorry. I've been busy fighting a war," I said semi-humorously.

"But the deadline was last week, and I was supposed to have handed them in to the Ministry of Education!"

"But I have been in the army for the past three and a half weeks, so I couldn't do it," I explained, scarcely able to believe that I was holding this conversation.

The dialog of the deaf continued:

"I tried and tried calling your home, but you were never there," he complained.

"Yes. I know. I was off fighting a war!"

"I even called your parents' home to look for you. But no success."

By this time, I was getting fed up.

"Mr. Bargur," I said in a peremptory voice, "When do you want the grades?"

"Now."

I went to the office, took a copy of the class list, and wrote down the grades as best as I could from memory. I made sure to give the students the benefit of the doubt. Mr. Bargur was finally happy, and the bureaucratic beast had been fed.

While I was at the school, I had further proof of the smallness of Israel with Jerusalem, in many ways, no more than a small village. All of a sudden, while I was talking to a group of students, one of them said: "We heard you are getting a citation." News certainly travels fast! I explained to them that I had been told that Dudu had *nominated* me, but that I probably would not get one. I was incredulous – how had they found out? I later learned that Yossie, my platoon commander, is the nephew of a professor at the University, and somehow the news had traveled next door to the high school.

As was bound to happen, one of the men in my platoon failed to show up to return to the platoon after his 24-hour leave, and so the next rifleman had to go back to the unit and was not able to go on leave that day. This is a very upsetting thing to happen when you are literally on your way home on leave, and we were all furious with him.

When he returned the following day, Dudu immediately placed the soldier on a charge and sentenced him to 14 days in military prison to begin the day we were discharged. We were shocked. Yes, we were furious because the guy who had come back a day late had caused such bitter disappointment to the soldier due for leave after him, but to sentence him to 14 days jail *after* we were finally to be discharged seemed to us excessive. We all gathered together in a room, closed the door and had a discussion as to what to do about this. It was decided that Dudu had to be approached and asked to change the punishment. And I was chosen to be the spokesperson. I was not at all happy about this assignment. After all, my Hebrew was not perfect, and in any case what we were doing was challenging the decision, and therefore the very authority, of a military officer. This was not a youth movement camp – this was the army, with all the requisite laws and regulations to back up any order. All I had going for me was that I knew Dudu to be a deeply thoughtful man, an exceptional leader, and I hoped he knew me to be a serious, honest person.

I approached Dudu and asked for an appointment to see him.

"Well, David, what is it?" he asked, when I came to the appointment. He did not have the first clue why I wanted to see him.

"Dudu, we in the platoon feel that the punishment you gave the man who came back a day late from leave is unfair," I explained as politely as I could.

"In what way unfair?" he asked. No rising anger, no defensiveness.

"We feel that what he did was very wrong, and that he deserves to be punished, but to sentence him to 14 days military prison, to begin *after* he has just finished about 4 weeks of service fighting a war, does not seem right."

"What are you asking me to do?" he asked quietly.

"We are asking you to reconsider and to alter the punishment."

I held my breath.

"What punishment would you suggest?"

"We thought you should give him an extra heavy load of guard duty and clean-up duty instead."

Again I held my breath.

"I think you are right. I will change the punishment," he said.

And so he did.

I described Dudu as a great human being, and this only reinforced my opinion. He was to demonstrate this same humanity and uniqueness of spirit again during the Yom Kippur War six years later.

After we had spent about a week in Bethlehem, our battalion fanned out southwards holding much of the southern area of what has come to be called 'the West Bank' between Bethlehem and Hebron. I personally spent the last part of this call up in a little village, El Chader, adjacent to Beit Jala, and a couple of kilometers west of Bethlehem. This was not a very eventful period – the Jordanian army had been severely mauled in the war, and there was no attempt on their part to counterattack or to regain any of the lost territory. They were truly in disarray. Nor, indeed, was there any trouble from the local Palestinian population. It is ironic now, as I write, to realize that at the time the term 'Palestinian' was not used for the Arabs of the West Bank. However, since today it is the term currently employed, I will use it to describe the West Bank and Gaza Arabs, even though the term is anachronistic. Jordan had had control of the West Bank since the end of the 1948 War of Independence, but had never allowed the Palestinians who fled there as refugees to integrate into Jordanian society – in some sense they were invisible to both sides.

Frankly, my impression was that the average Palestinian civilian was traumatized, and understandably so. After all, their side had lost the war, and now they were being occupied by the very army which – so their propaganda had constantly warned them – was a brutal force, greatly to be feared. So although we had to be on our guard and careful, of course, I would even describe this period as boring – we spent most of our time guarding, going out on patrols and sleeping.

Finally, some four to five weeks after having been called up, we were discharged. And what a thrill that was. But, attached to our discharge papers was a call up paper summoning us to another four weeks of *miluim* a month later in what we then referred to as the 'liberated territories' (i.e., the West Bank). When that time came, the additional month was not very different from the period after we arrived in Bethlehem. We were all eager to tour the West Bank and Gaza, and so our officers arranged whole-day tours of the entire area, which was still under military control and closed to the public; we, of course, were allowed to travel around freely as we were part of the force serving in the area. Six or seven soldiers accompanied by a *chovesh* and an officer would set off on these one-day trips in army command cars. At first this was exciting, but because we medics had to be included, and there were not many of us, the novelty soon wore off, as we were instructed to go on this circular trip of the whole West Bank sometimes day after day. Command cars are not the best sprung or upholstered vehicles in the world, and a picnic lunch of battle ration tinned food held little appeal either.

One day we were told that our wives could come and spend the day with us – they were to be picked up in the centre of Jerusalem, and brought by army truck to where we were serving. This was still a restricted military area, so it was exciting for them as civilians to have this opportunity, and of course a treat for us to see them for the day. They had been told to bring a picnic lunch. We were full of anticipation – it was all a little reminiscent of visiting day for prisoners! The previous evening, one of the sergeants, Yishai, came to me and informed me that I was the medic going on the 'West Bank tour' the following morning.

"I cannot go – my wife is coming with the group of wives to spend the day with me."

"We have no other medic available, so you will have to go," he said.

"But she'll arrive with the truck, not find me here, and, what is more, she'll be stuck here for the whole day."

Suddenly Yishai had an idea: "Has your wife ever toured the West Bank?" he asked.

"Never."

"Well how about this: the command car going on the tour will drive to your apartment, pick her up, and she will do the tour with you. We

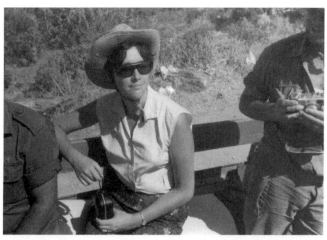

Jenny "disguised" as a soldier, touring the West Bank, June 1967.

will take an army shirt and hat with us for her to wear so that the Military Police at the roadblocks don't give us any trouble."

Knowing Jenny to be a real sport I thought that this was a wonderful solution, and was confident that she would be in full and enthusiastic agreement, too. So, the following morning, very early, we drove into Jerusalem, and the entire group waited in the command car while I ran upstairs to my parents' apartment where once again Jenny was staying, woke her and told her to get dressed quickly as she was going on a tour of the West Bank. Jenny put the army shirt on top of her own shirt, donned the army hat, and off we went. We dropped her back late that afternoon. We had had a marvelously happy day together enjoying each other's company, with Jenny getting her first glimpse of the West Bank. Apart from anything else, after riding in a military transport she had now acquired a heightened appreciation of the upholstery and springs on our own family car!

After this additional month's service, we were discharged for the second time, and were greatly relieved to return to civilian life – this time for real. But times were to get worse quite soon, and little did we know that there would be a huge amount of *miluim* waiting for us in the next several years. Maybe the old joke that an Israeli citizen is an Israeli soldier on eleven months' leave is not such a joke after all.

In those heady days after the sweeping victory by *Tzahal*, Jenny and I – and, in fact, many Israelis – were inundated with visitors from abroad. Friends and family just poured in – some had come as volunteers, and some arrived on visits after the victory. These not only included Steve, heading a group of South African volunteers, but also Jenny's brother, Leon, who by this time had left Israel and gone to live in Britain. They all wanted to tour the West Bank and Gaza so, as soon as the area was opened to the civilian public, we found ourselves doing the Grand Tour on eight consecutive Saturdays. By then, having also done it several times in the army, I was desperately tired of it – but our visitors, of course, were not.

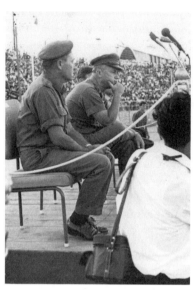

Yitzchak Rabin, our Commander-in-Chief, reviewing us as we marched past in the Victory Parade.

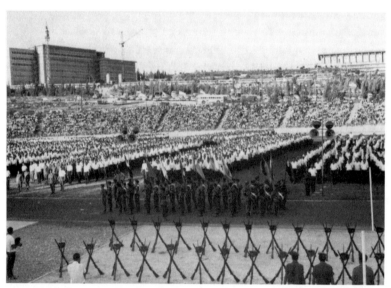

Victory Parade of the Jerusalem Brigade, held at Givat Ram shortly after the Six Day War. The rifles support helmets, each of which contains a flame representing one of the fallen.

A couple of months after we were demobilized there was a Victory Parade of our Brigade in the stadium of the Hebrew University. A flame was burning in upended helmets supported by rifles in the 'piled arms' position, one for each soldier from the brigade who had been killed in the war A most moving sight. Virtually every one of us was a reservist, with the exception of the battalion commanders and a few other higher ranks, and we all marched past the saluting platform with great pride. As we had all been discharged we marched past, not in uniform, but in white shirts and black pants. The salute was taken by the Commander-in-Chief, Yitzchak Rabin. As much as I keep referring to myself as a reluctant soldier, I was extremely emotional and proud that day. I had been a part of the liberation of Jerusalem, and had played a part in saving my home and my family and, indeed, my very country.

But the pride and euphoria that we all felt at that moment soon began to dissipate, at least for Jenny and me. It quickly became evident to us that the military occupation of the West Bank and Gaza was wrong, and that no biblical or historical imperative could justify keeping a people in subjugation. In fact, not only were we keeping the people who lived on the West Bank in subjugation, but Israel started to find itself imprisoned in the role of conqueror and occupier, rapidly developing new settlements and suburbs across the old border to establish 'facts on the ground' before any possible peace treaty.

Yeshayahu Leibowitz, an elderly professor of philosophy at the Hebrew University, wrote a few months after the war that this military occupation must end – that it was like a cancer that would eat into the very fiber of our society. And that is precisely how Jenny and I felt. But we were a minority, and Israel was not only giddy with victory, but chose to adopt an arrogant stance and did not, in my opinion, press hard enough for peace.

This feeling of discomfort over the continuing occupation and the building of Jewish settlements in the West Bank remained with us, and indeed remains with us to this very day. This does not alter the fact that even greater responsibility for what has transpired in the past fifty-five years rests with the Arabs of the surrounding states. Ever since the creation of the State of Israel in 1948, the Arabs have not only not sought peace with Israel but have fought to destroy it. They have kept the Palestinians as refugees in camps, preferring to employ them as political pawns instead of working to make them productive, integrated members of their societies, as Israel has done with the vast number of refugees that have arrived since 1948. It is a little remembered fact that as many Jews left Arab lands around 1948 and came to Israel as Arabs left Israel to become refugees on the West Bank.

And so the Six Day War period, an extraordinary chapter in Israel's history, came to an end. It was no less momentous a period in my own life – six years earlier, still a boy, I'd just arrived from South Africa, knowing no one in this new land. As we returned to civilian life, and as Jenny and I and our families went back to our regular routines and our lives resumed their normal courses, everything seemed the same, and indeed on a day-to-day basis it was – but on a national level something fundamental had occurred, which was to change the face and destiny of Israel forever.

Part III

*BETWEEN THE SIX DAY WAR
AND THE OUTBREAK OF
THE YOM KIPPUR WAR*

The period from the end of the Six Day War to the outbreak of the Yom Kippur War six years later was militarily a much more turbulent one for me than my earlier periods of reserve duty, and this came as quite a shock. As a result of the Six Day War, all *miluimniks* now had to perform a greatly increased number of days of service each year guarding and patrolling the huge areas of land, many times its own size, which had come under Israeli rule: the entire West Bank and Gaza, plus the whole of the Sinai peninsula. All of this had to be administered and guarded, and that required large numbers of soldiers and with every group, without exception, a *chovesh*.

During this period between "my" two wars, I was called up to do a more advanced medic's course. This time, it was in order to become a *chovesh ta'agad* – the next step up the military promotion ladder – a medic who worked with the battalion doctor in the Battalion Aid Station. While each platoon and company has a medic, behind them is the *ta'agad*, serving a whole battalion. A *ta'agad* is staffed by a doctor, a radio man, and six to eight more highly trained medics, and is equipped with an ambulance and much more sophisticated medical supplies than platoon medics carried or knew how to use.

The original course that I did in 1964 was the shortest course offered by the Medical Corps, since it was given as part of reserve, rather than of national, service. Consequently we had received minimal training and the army, quite correctly, felt that we needed additional instruction and practice. Furthermore, by 1969, Israel had learned from the American experience in Vietnam that if every medic carried bags of fluid and was trained to insert an IV with fluids to replace lost blood, many lives could be saved. It had been shown that the sooner the supply of replacement fluids began, the greater the chance of saving the injured soldier's life.

As before, I really enjoyed the course because it was intensely interesting and we learned a great deal, including how to insert IVs and how to give injections. The course's highlight for me was a week's work in the Emergency Department of a large civilian hospital, in my case Hadassah hospital in Jerusalem. Here, among other things, the staff – happy to let us get as much practice as we could – made sure to call us to insert an IV whenever one was needed.

The period between 1967 and 1973 was that of the 'War of Attrition' with Egypt, in which *Tzahal* and the Egyptian Army shelled each other constantly across the Suez Canal, and the cost in lives on both sides and property damage, for example in the town of Suez, was enormous. Even more important, this was also the period of active terrorism from across the Jordanian border to Israel's east. A large part of the border was now marked by the Jordan River, which flows from the southern extremity of the Sea of Galilee southwards to the northern tip of the Dead Sea. The Palestinians are Arabs, many of whom now live in Jordan, but most of whose parents or grandparents lived in what is today Israel or the Israeli-occupied West Bank, and who were displaced from their homes by the wars with Israel. They provided a ready source of recruits for groups such as the Fatah movement headed by Yasser Arafat, which had as its aim the liberation of Palestine and which was principally responsible for the considerable amount of quite serious terrorist activity from across the Jordan River. There were casualties each day both here and along the Suez Canal front, and we used to turn on the radio to hear the news with a horrible sense of foreboding. These casualties were often *miluimniks* like myself, and when units like mine went off to do a stint of service, it was anything but sure that all of us would return. The particularly bad period on the Jordanian border lasted from about 1968 until September 1970. At that point, King Hussein of Jordan, a Hashemite Bedouin and not a Palestinian, realized that the presence and actions of the Fatah were destabilizing his country and threatening his monarchy. Accordingly he attacked Fatah, killing many and driving the remainder, under Arafat's leadership, out of Jordan and into Lebanon in a bitterly fought action which has come to be known as 'Black September.'

During this period, my *miluim* was mainly on the Jordanian border – in the Jordan Valley, or along the Jordan River. However, I did also serve one term in the Sinai and one on the Golan Heights.

All eligible Israelis inevitably found that, in this period between the two wars, *miluim* played a great role in their lives. The call ups were invariably for a longer period than I had been accustomed to before the Six Day War, and often lasted as long as six weeks. Moreover, the very nature of the service changed. Whereas most *miluim* before 1967 consisted of exercises and of practicing different maneuvers, after 1967 things were quite different. Sometimes it would begin with the *chovshim* spending two to three days doing an intensive refresher course in First Aid before the rest of the unit arrived. Then, once the unit was fully assembled, we usually spent four to six days doing intensive training and maneuvers, and then were sent to guard different outposts, usually along the Jordan River. This was real 'active service,' and we came to learn the full implications of the term.

The specific period of *miluim* I am about to describe occurred at the end of 1968. We reported for duty in the full knowledge that this was going to be serious and dangerous. After all, each of us followed the news closely, and also knew friends in parallel units who had served in this area, so were perfectly well aware what lay in store for us. We did the usual period of training, which I always hated, as it involved infantry exercises consisting of running up and down hills and going on long marches, struggling all the while with the mass of medical equipment that *chovshim* had to carry in addition to their standard infantry packs. And what had been heavy grew heavier still: ever since *chovshim* were taught to insert IVs, six one-liter bags of fluid were added to the already weighty equipment we were required to carry.

At the end of the exercises we were divided up and sent to different outposts (*mutzavim*) along the Jordan River. *Mutzavim* were dotted all along the Jordanian border, and groups of soldiers manned each one. The way it worked was that the newcomers who were replacing the *miluimniks* who were just finishing their term spent 24 hours together, so that the old-timers could demonstrate everything that needed to be shown to their replacements who were shadowing them. (It is known as 'overlap' or 'chafifa' in military jargon.) Our night of *chafifa* was enough to tell me that I did not much like what I was going to be doing. The outgoing *chovesh* whom I shadowed told me that there had not been a night that there had not been shooting in both directions, and that it was very dangerous, very cold, and very uncomfortable. What a perfectly delightful combination!

We defended the outpost with guards facing in all directions, not just eastwards towards Jordan, in case infiltrators managed to get across the river and come at us from the rear or the flanks. This had indeed happened right where we were stationed just a couple of months earlier, when two infiltrators had managed to penetrate the outpost from the rear, killing two soldiers from our brigade before they themselves were killed. It must be borne in mind that even in this wintry, rainy season, the Jordan River was hardly a serious barrier. At the place where we were located it was shallow enough to be able to wade through – the water did not nearly reach waist height, and the Jordan is remarkably narrow, a mere stream and nothing like its depiction in the spirituals I used to sing in Habonim. As there was always the danger of infiltrators, our defensive strategy called for us to guard and sleep in the same place. No one moved in the *mutzav* after dark, since it was just too perilous for us to be walking around inside the perimeter at night lest we be mistaken for infiltrators. We guarded in pairs in trenches that were a little lower than waist height, and running off them at right angles to the guard trench were what were known as 'shfaniyot,' or 'rabbit hutches.' These were little tunnels, just short of six feet long, about two feet wide and about eighteen inches high. They were covered with sandbags, and that is where we slept when it was not our turn to guard – you had to crawl into the rabbit hutch as best you could, and go to sleep right there, next to the feet of the people who were on guard duty. There were two choices: You could go in headfirst, and that was the warmer way, but it was also stifling in there. Alternatively, you could go in feet first, but then, dependent on your height, there was a danger – certainly true in my case – of your head sticking out into the trench and being trodden on. The loveliest aspect of all was that the rabbit hutch was too low to turn over in or to lie on your side. As you can imagine, such sleeping arrangements did not give rise to the term 'beauty sleep.' Being right there with the guards also guaranteed that you would be disturbed – either by being inadvertently kicked, or by the guards whispering amongst themselves, or by sudden bursts of small arms fire.

I was stationed at the front of the *mutzav* facing eastwards across the Jordan River, with my platoon commander, Yossie, the same Yossie

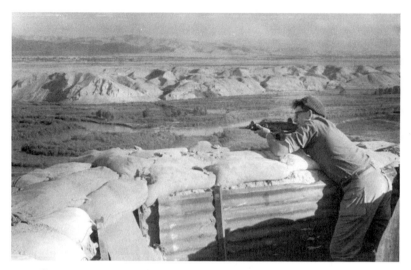

Guarding in a mutzav *on the banks of the Jordan River, 1969.*

who had been my platoon commander during the Six Day War. In fact, we often guarded together. I had come to know him well, and he me, and we got on famously together. A decent man, I think a little younger than I was, and a very fine soldier who had won my respect in the Six Day War. However, he was not one of those officers whom one would ever call a *chevreman*, or fun guy. When it came to military matters, Yossie was deadly serious and always played it by the book

Almost every night there were bursts of light arms and mortar fire either aimed directly at us or occurring near us. On one particular night, during the time that I was in my rabbit hutch and not guarding, there was a particularly serious exchange of fire, and all of a sudden I felt someone kicking my feet. (I had gone in headfirst to get warm.) It was Yossie.

"Get up. There's a major incident developing," he shouted.

I was very angry to have been wakened. I'd managed to stay asleep through all of the shooting and shelling, proving how one can get used to anything. On that particular occasion, although the firing was heavier than usual, it did not in fact turn into a major incident but, like so many situations in military life proved, much to my relief, to be a false alarm.

Thank goodness we managed to get through our time in that *mutzav* without anyone being injured. But that was not true for the whole line. While I was at that *mutzav* some Fatah infiltrators managed to get across the line a little south of us near Jericho, and they were not stopped before two officers had been killed. One of them was a high ranking and well known soldier who, it was rumored, was being groomed for the position of chief of staff.

Injury and fatalities were commonplace. Jenny and I were to learn just how commonplace all too soon. An example of what went on occurred just a couple of months before my term at this *mutzav*. Another *miluim* unit had been guarding the same *mutzav*, and one of their soldiers was very seriously injured in an exchange of fire. That soldier was guarding the rear. In other words, if the *mutzav* faced east towards Jordan, this man was facing west in case there was infiltration from the rear. The corporal at the rear radioed to the platoon commander at the front of the *mutzav* that they needed the *chovesh* urgently – that it was a matter of life and death. The platoon commander thought quickly, and informed all the guard posts that he was sending the *chovesh* clockwise to the back, and no one was to shoot him. If you imagine a clock with the platoon commander stationed at twelve o'clock, he sent the *chovesh* to the six o'clock position via the three o'clock position.

It was pitch dark, the shooting and shelling was continuous, everyone was desperately tense, and everyone knew that there were serious injuries to some of their comrades. The *chovesh* himself was no less tense and scared, and inadvertently set out in a counter-clockwise direction. He was just reaching the nine o'clock position, when those soldiers saw someone approaching, knew it could not be one of their soldiers as they did not move around the *mutzav* after dark, and opened fire with automatic weapons, killing their own *chovesh* instantly. The critically injured soldier he was to have attended also died, unattended, of his wounds.

But it was not always as terrible as that, and during my stint we escaped without anyone being injured. During the day, apart from shifts of guard duty, we were relatively free to sleep, play ping pong in a prefabricated hut in the center of the *mutzav*, eat, write letters, or read.

Eating, in fact, became something of a preoccupation for us in our cramped quarters, with the cook doing a superb job creating what we came to regard as gourmet meals for us – making the most of the supplies with which he was provided. The cook was one of us from the platoon, and not a professional, working at preparing meals in lieu of some other duties. Basically, he used the rations supplied by the army, which were not too bad as we had refrigeration facilities and could therefore keep fresh produce. And then he would augment what the army gave him with some spices that he brought from home. He was a real genius in the kitchen and was the unchallenged hero of the group. As lunchtime approached, we would all gravitate to the kitchen area and hover until the meal was ready. He and I were on particularly good terms, and sometimes he would even make dishes that I specially requested such as my favorite, a good beef stew with french fries.

Of course we could not leave the *mutzav* except when it was our turn to go on leave. Whoever returned from leave had first to make his way back to our headquarters, and then from there be driven to the *mutzav*. They were always given the mail – our lifeline – to bring from headquarters. One day, Ronen, who had just got back from leave, came up to me and said, "Hit me, David. Hit me hard."

"Why should I?"

"Just hit me, please."

After refusing again, I demanded that he explain. He told me that he had collected the mail to bring to us as usual, but a postcard from Jenny had blown out of his hand in the open command car and come to rest in a minefield.

"How do you know it was from my wife?" I asked.

"Because I read it," he admitted sheepishly. "And she's fine and so are your parents and they all send love."

What could I say?

There were four things we lived for while doing this kind of service: the meals, leave, phone calls from home, and the end of the tour of duty. I have already mentioned the efforts of our cook, how highly he was esteemed and how much we valued the fruits of his labor and ingenuity. But leave.... Now that was truly precious! When *miluim* begins, you are informed how many people can be away at once, and for how long. As always, there was a special rule for *chovshim*. In keeping with the regulation that every unit had to have a *chovesh* at all times, we were only allowed to go on leave when a replacement arrived. My turn eventually came, and I spent a couple of glorious days at home. Jenny was working, of course, and could not always get time off, but still it was wonderful to be with her and to see my parents. Being a *miluimnik* on leave was totally unremarkable, since so many men were in *miluim* so often. I spent most of my time at home, visiting the school where I taught, visiting Jenny's and my mother's offices (my father did not like being disturbed at work) and just relaxing.

One time, while I was at home, I got stomach flu and was not feeling too well the day I returned but, of course, still had to rejoin my unit. In any case, I was simply feeling a little queasy, and wasn't by any means seriously ill. That very night, when we were already in our guard positions, we learned over the field telephone that we were being patched through to the army telephone exchange in order to be able to speak with our families. Getting a chance to call home was rare. It was always a thrilling moment, and I was excited even though I had left Jenny just that morning. Of course, it would have been much better had this connection been made during the day, but it was precious and not to be wasted.

We took it in turns speaking, but Yossie made it crystal clear to us that we were to whisper. We were only a few hundred meters from the border, and could easily be heard in the quiet of the night. When my turn came, I expectantly gave my number to the military telephonist and waited while she dialed.

Finally I heard Jenny's lovely voice, "Hello."

"Hello, Jen," I whispered.

"Who is this?" Jenny, worried.

"It's me, David."

"What's wrong? Are you ill?" Jenny asked, in an even more anxious voice.

And then I realized what was going on: I was whispering, and she had said goodbye to me that morning knowing I was not feeling one hundred percent, whereupon she put two and two together and got twenty two! I quickly clarified that I was fine but that, for "certain reasons," I had to whisper. Jenny understood, and the two of us burst out laughing.

The fourth thing we lived for was the day when it would all be over and we could go home. Every day we would cross off the previous day on the calendar and announce how many more days there were still to go. This is somewhat reminiscent, surely, of what prisoners serving time do in prison.

The particular *miluim* I have been describing included New Year's Eve. On that day I was very 'down.' New Year's Eve is our wedding anniversary, and being apart was awful. Jenny and I had got married, in Jerusalem, four years earlier, and the army was keeping us apart on our anniversary. Needless to say, this was not grounds for not serving and we could do nothing about it, but we were entitled to be sad. Jenny and I have always treated our anniversary as a very special day, and we never fail to try to do something exciting. Not this time.

We always guarded in pairs, and that night, as I was standing guard, I had an idea. I went over to Yossie, with whom I was again paired, and whispered the following proposal to him:

"At the stroke of midnight, let's fire off a mortar flare to herald the new year," I proposed.

"On no account!" was the straight-laced Yossie's prim response. "These flares are only to be used for military purposes when we suspect something suspicious."

Whenever there was any suspicion of an infiltration, we would fire off a flare from a mortar to light up the area. These flares would light up the dark night sky with an eerie but bright light for a good thirty seconds, or maybe even a little more, and this enabled us to determine whether anyone was indeed approaching. It was always a little scary to fire them off, as we did not know what we would find, but it was also comforting to be able to see the terrain clearly. Yossie, as platoon commander, was allowed to fire off as many flares as he needed, and the supply would be replenished in the morning.

"Oh, come on, Yossie. It's not only New Year's Eve, but it is also my wedding anniversary," I pleaded.

After much thought he replied, "Okay, I'll do it!"

The plan was that Yossie would prepare the flare for firing, and I would listen to the radio with my ear-plug so as to know the exact time and, at the stroke of midnight, I would signal to Yossie and he would fire off the flare. We felt like naughty schoolboys.

There I was, ear-plug in ear, Yossie with his hand on the mortar ready to fire the flare, and the countdown to midnight on *Kol Yisrael* (The Voice of Israel) Radio began: Ten-nine-eight-seven- six (I raised my hand) – five-four-three-two-one, and I lowered my hand. Yossie fired off the flare. And suddenly we saw what was happening: as far as the eye could see, northwards and southwards up and down the border, every *mutzav* had done the same thing! We burst out laughing uncontrollably. I often wonder what the Fatah thought was happening at that moment.

During another period of *miluim* in which we were again stationed in a *mutzav*, we also went out on patrols along the Jordan River bank every night. This meant that there was not only danger from the Jordanian forces, but even more serious was the presence of Fatah terrorists who tried nightly to infiltrate and attack the *Tzahal* units, usually by ambush. What made the patrols so dangerous was that we did not patrol quietly in darkened vehicles, but on the contrary patrolled in armored troop carriers that had floodlights strung above them, so that we looked a little like a circus vehicle or a Superbowl float approaching. The idea was to announce to the Jordanians and to Arafat's Fatah that we were in control of this area, and that they should not try anything. But, as you can imagine, this also made us perfect targets for terrorists lying in ambush waiting for our 'parade.' The tension on these patrols was enormous, and for their duration no one said a word – we simply rode along in silence, trying to scan the bush for possible infiltrators.

During this period of *miluim*, a new soldier was added to our strength at our *mutzav*. We were told that he was a pacifist. He had no sooner arrived than he announced that he refused to carry a weapon on principle. The officer in charge was smart, and made no attempt to try and argue with him.

"No problem," he said. "Just put your rifle carefully under your bed. But be sure to report on time for this evening's patrol along the border. And that's an order."

That evening the new soldier duly reported for the patrol, and rode with us on the armored troop carrier, unarmed. He must have been every bit as terrified as I was. The following evening he reported for the patrol, didn't say a word, but this time had his rifle with him, and that was the end of the problem. I am, I confess, a little ashamed to say that we were not particularly nice to this guy, and treated him as an outcast because of his behavior, which was endangering all our lives as well as his own.

When not on *miluim* and leading my civilian life, I continued working at the Hebrew University High School. Here I made several friends among the teachers, particularly among the English teachers who were the ones with whom I worked most intimately. Three of these teachers, with whom Jenny and I became close friends, were Gilda and Marion, both new immigrants from the United States and both single at this time, and Nadav, a *Sabra*, that is to say someone born in Israel. That friendship was to lead me to one of the most heartbreaking experiences of my life.

I quickly became friendly with Nadav. He was bright, delightful, fun and, as all my female students used constantly to remind me, exceptionally good looking. Nadav was the *Gadna* instructor at the school. *Gadna* is the pre-service paramilitary cadet organization that is intended to prepare high school students for their army service. The *Gadna* instructors were responsible for preparing the students mentally by teaching them civics, and physically by taking them on hikes and other physically taxing outings in order to make them fit. Nadav had attended a military high school in his native Haifa, and had reached the rank of lieutenant during his national service.

We, their circle of friends, were all delighted when a romance began to blossom between Nadav and Marion. Marion was attractive, vivacious, fun loving, witty and most appealing. We all thought this a great match, although I am not sure the girls at the school would have entirely agreed, because many of them were reported to be infatuated with Nadav and horribly envious of Marion. Time passed, and eventually Nadav and Marion married early in 1968. Naturally we were all thrilled, and our friendship continued, growing ever more intimate.

Nadav and I became particularly close when he led a five day camping trip to the Negev desert and to Eilat, Israel's Red Sea port; I was one of the accompanying teachers on this outing. We were short staffed, and were responsible for supervising four eleventh-grade classes, so we really had our hands full. What made it all so difficult was that here we were, with some 120 eleventh-graders, camped on the shores of the Red Sea, with a strict and explicit ruling by the principal of the school, Dr. Shamir, that no one was to be allowed to swim. While this ruling may sound peculiar in the extreme, in fairness to Dr. Shamir allowing a group of youngsters to swim is a huge responsibility which he, rightly or wrongly, was unwilling for the school to assume. There were also issues of lifeguarding and insurance liability. To keep them all out of the water all of the time was well nigh impossible, and attempting to do so required some smart teamwork on the part of Nadav, myself and the couple of other adults with us. When we finally managed to get all those hyperactive seventeen-year olds into their pup tents at night, Nadav and I would heave a sigh of mingled relief and exhaustion, then collapse into our own tent. Here we'd chat about all sorts of things as we unwound after a grueling day of hiking and an even more grueling night of chasing after students. However everyone had a fine time, and we all returned home safely. Nadav and I had worked well together, and by the end of the trip had become really close.

Now at about this time I had applied for a British Council Scholarship to go to Britain for a year to do an M.A. in Applied Linguistics, since Israel did not then have such a program. The Israeli M.A. programs covered some of the areas I was interested in, but they were not comparable with what was being offered in Britain. Moreover, had I done my M.A. in Israel, I would have been unlikely to receive any financial assistance, and would have had to do it part time while working. The British Council Scholarship, on the other hand, would cover my travel, tuition, accommodation and food for the entire year, so that I would be able to devote all my time to my studies. Much to my delight I was awarded the scholarship, and the British Council secured a place for me in the Master's program at the University of Wales in

Bangor, North Wales. It involved a nine month academic year of coursework followed by the writing of a thesis, which I planned to do during the three summer months following the end of the program. Jenny and I decided to take our car with us to Britain, and planned to sail by ferry to Piraeus in Greece, then drive all the way from there, touring Europe as we went. More or less concurrent with getting the news that I had won the scholarship, we learned that Jenny was pregnant and expecting in November.

We were looking forward to our year overseas for another reason as well, since it would give us the perspective of distance to enable us to assess how our lives were developing, and indeed how the country itself was developing, too. For although Israel at this point had returned to normal after the upheaval caused by the 1967 war, as far as Jenny and I were concerned it was not 'business as usual.' We were becoming increasingly disturbed by the policies of successive governments, who steadfastly adhered to a policy of building settlements on the West Bank and in Gaza, blithely and arrogantly ignoring the protestations of the Arab residents of the area. As early as this we had begun to toy with the idea of emigrating, but that was as far as it went.

Very shortly after hearing the good news of the scholarship, we discovered that Marion and Nadav were going to the U.S. that same summer to visit Marion's parents, who had continued to live there rather than follow their daughter to Israel. We hit on an idea. Jenny and I would take the ferry to Greece with the car, while Nadav and Marion would fly later to Zurich where we would all meet on a pre-arranged date in July and tour Switzerland together. Nadav and Marion would then fly to the U.S., and Jenny and I would continue on our way to Britain.

Mid-June, 1969. The weather was getting warm, and the school year was finally coming to an end. We were just two weeks away from our eagerly anticipated trip with Nadav and Marion. School began at 8.00 a.m., and Dr. Shamir was *extremely* strict about us getting to class immediately the bell rang. He did not accept excuses for lateness, and was often in the corridors checking up on us, the teachers, as much as on the students. The bell rang, and as I was leaving the staff room for class, I was called to the internal telephone. It was the principal.

"Come up to my office immediately," he barked.

"But the bell has rung and I have a class."

"Never mind the class – I'll send someone to cover for you. You come up to my office right away."

I realized something important, something unusual, something vaguely disquieting was taking place.

I knocked at his door, and on entering found the principal, the vice-principal, Mr.Bargur the school secretary, and a man in army uniform, all looking very somber. My heart sank.

"Where is Marion?" the principal asked.

"I have no idea. I didn't see her in the staff room. Did you check her schedule?" I asked.

"She doesn't teach until later in the day, and she's not at home," he said.

"What has happened?" I pleaded. "Please tell me. Something is clearly wrong."

All four men looked at the floor.

"Marion is one of my closest friends. *Please* tell me."

"Nadav has fallen. (This is the Hebrew euphemism for describing a soldier who has been killed in action.) He was killed in *miluim* last night while leading a patrol along the Jordan River. They were ambushed by Fatah guerillas."

I began to shake.

The man in army uniform was from the Town Major's office (*Katzin Ha'ir*), the members of which are required, as one of their duties, to go to the family of a soldier who has been killed and break the news. He had duly gone to Nadav and Marion's apartment to tell her, but there was no one there, so he had come to her place of work.

"Marion often sleeps over with friends when Nadav is in *miluim*," I explained. "But she may well have returned home by now."

At that moment there was a knock at the door. It was Gilda. She, too, had been summoned. After a few moments, they broke the news to her. She was shattered.

The *Katzin Ha'ir* decided that he wanted to go back to the apartment to see if Marion had returned in the meantime, and he asked Gilda and me if we would accompany him. After all, Marion had no family in Israel, and he felt that she would need the support of close friends. Of course we agreed.

This was a new role for both of us, one I never want to have to repeat.

We walked through the courtyard of their apartment complex, and as we did people opened their doors to watch where this 'Angel of Death' in *Tzahal* uniform was heading. *They* knew only too well what his grim presence meant. Sadly, with the history that it has, they knew that this was the way it was done in *Tzahal* – not by telegram, like in all the Second World War movies.

We rang the bell, and Marion came to the door. She was busy hanging the laundry.

"Are you Marion?" the officer asked.

"Yes," she replied.

"Please sit down."

Marion did so.

"I am afraid I have bad news. Nadav has fallen. He was leading a patrol along the Jordan border last night, and they were ambushed."

Marion remained silent for a moment, stunned, and then said, "I must go to Haifa, to his parents."

"I'll drive you," I said.

"It's not necessary," she protested. " I'll take the bus." This was typical Marion – never wanting to put anybody out, not even at a time like this. Marion is a slightly built woman, and at that moment, despite the enormous strength that it took to respond in the way she did, she looked very small and very vulnerable.

Of course we did not allow her to take the bus. Gilda and I took it in turns to rush home to gather up some clothes for ourselves as we realized that the funeral would be in Haifa the following day, and that we would be staying over. Gilda also made a thermos of hot tea for us to take in the car. By that time another close friend, Shula, had arrived, and she too accompanied us to Haifa.

I will never forget that trip. Gilda, Shula, Marion and I drove for close to three hours in absolute silence. No tears, no talk of what a wonderful person Nadav was. Just silence.

This was 1969, and the roads were not nearly as good as they are today. The journey seemed endless. What is more, the *Katzin Ha'ir* had asked us to call him from the outskirts of Haifa to ensure that they had already broken the news to Nadav's parents before we arrived at their home. This required a stop at a gas station (this was the pre-mobile phone era) and, on the pretext of needing the men's room, I left the car, found a pay phone and confirmed that the parents had been informed. We were also careful about turning on the radio. We knew that they would be announcing the incident on the news every hour, and we worried that Marion would become distraught on hearing Nadav's name, so we managed to work it that the radio was never on at the hour, and we always seemed 'to just miss' the news.

We drove to Nadav's parents' apartment, and the scene on our arrival was nothing short of heartbreaking, with Nadav's parents hugging their daughter-in-law, Marion, and sobbing. She and Nadav had only been married for about 18 months.

At the apartment was Adam, Nadav's best friend from the days when they had attended the military high school academy together. Adam had been born in South Africa, and I discovered that his oldest brother had been in my class for six months in high school before their family emigrated to Israel. While the army did the logistical planning of the funeral and in effect made all the arrangements, these still had to be coordinated with the immediate family, none of whom understandably was in a fit state to take care of it. So Adam and I did. Moreover, the funeral had to be delayed long enough to allow Marion's parents time to arrive from the United States.

Nadav received a military burial. This was not the first I had attended, as I'd been involved in a couple of the funerals of the people in my company killed in the Six Day War, but none was nearly as close to me as Nadav was. It was just heart-rending. Two days after he fell we buried Nadav in the Haifa military cemetery, and Marion spent the *shiva* week in Haifa with her in-laws. A sign-up sheet went up at the school immediately, and every day of the *shiva* at least one car-load –

and often two – set off for Haifa to condole with Marion and with Nadav's family. Sad to say, that is the kind of thing that Israelis do so well.

Eight months later, reading an Israeli paper while in Britain, I learned that Adam, who had been of such signal help in the preparations for Nadav's funeral, had also been killed in *miluim*. And then Adam's younger brother, Gideon, was subsequently killed in the Yom Kippur War. Adam's and Gideon's parents were destroyed. And so the dreadful toll mounted.

Just around the time of Nadav's death, Jenny was advised that, because of her pregnancy, she should not take the long car trip we had planned across Europe. So I sailed to Venice and then drove from Venice to Amsterdam alone, where I met Jenny and we proceeded together to North Wales. As I drove across Europe I could not help but reflect that this solitary and mournful journey was a far cry indeed from the joyful trip envisaged in our planning with Nadav and Marion.

In November our eldest child Karen Lee was born in Bangor, North Wales, so when we returned to Israel a year later, I with my M.A. in hand, we had become a family of three, with another daughter, Noa, on the way. This had been a wonderful year in every way, and we had thoroughly enjoyed living on the island of Anglesey in rural Wales, utterly different in so many ways from our life in Israel. A few weeks after our return we had the joy of attending the wedding of Jenny's sister Beverley to Amichai, a celebration which they had kindly delayed pending our return. Amichai has served as an officer in the army and in *miluim* for years, and only a few years ago was finally discharged from all further duty. However, the inexorable cycle of Israeli life continues: Avi, his son, is now poised to begin his national service.

I had resigned from Hebrew University High School when we left for Britain, as I had been promised a position at the Hebrew University on my return, a post that I took up while Jenny resumed her position at the library. I was sad to leave the school, as I had been very happy there and had really grown to love the students. But the prospect of teaching at university was most exciting, and it offered tantalizing opportunities for advancement. I was in charge of the language laboratories, and my teaching was in the Linguistics section of the English Department; I felt almost as if I were among old friends, as many of my own professors in the department were still on faculty.

On a sadder note, we returned to confirm for ourselves what Jenny's mother had warned us of when she visited us in Anglesey – that 'something was wrong' and that my father's speech had become a little slurred. This had come as a terrible shock to us, all the more so as we were far from home and unable to provide immediate practical help to my parents.

Attitudes in the Israel to which we returned were even more entrenched, and there was very little serious talk of vacating the occupied territories or of stopping building new settlements. People were ambivalent about them – on the one hand they were said to be there to provide security for Israel, but on the other hand it was clear to us that their presence was not only wrong but that they were like a red rag to a bull for the Palestinians. And on the Palestinian side, indeed from the whole Arab camp, there was a deafening silence – no talk of peace whatsoever. We were deeply distressed as well as profoundly depressed by this lamentable state of affairs. Even *Tzahal* itself was affected, being now compelled to function, in the British phrase, 'in support of the civil power,' in other words acting as a subsidiary police force as much as an army of defense. Many of its actions now consisted simply of enforcing the occupation on the civilian Arab population of the occupied territories. Because of this, I was not sorry when I learned that my first *miluim* after our return was to be at Abu Rodez on the Gulf of Suez in Sinai, and not on the West Bank or, worse still, in Gaza. The down side was that the period of the *miluim* spanned December 1970-January 1971, meaning yet another wedding anniversary away from Jenny. Unlike previous *miluim*, we now we had a daughter, and it was not that easy to move her and Jenny and all her equipment to my parents' tiny place, so Jenny did not move in with them as she had done in the past. My father was still in pretty good health, and he and my mother took wonderful care of her: either they went after work every day to help her with baby Lee, or she went to my parents. In both cases my mother prepared most of the meals, helped bath and change the baby, and she and my father were always ready to baby-sit Lee. A deep love had grown between Jenny and my parents, and nothing they could do for her was ever too much trouble. Jenny, for her part, was a supremely attentive and loving daughter-in-law, caring and cooking for them and doing all the household chores whenever the tables were turned, as they eventually were as my father became more and more needy.

Abu Rodez is the place where the Egyptians had found oil, and after 1967 Israel was very busy pumping it out. Our main task was to guard the installations and civilian workers in the oil fields. Militarily the area was quiet and our days boring and monotonously uneventful, consisting of patrols, guard duty and simply being there for any eventuality.

The whole of the Sinai Peninsula was under military government at the time, and so there was no civilian authority in the area. This meant that the army was responsible for everything that went on there and, consequently, our medical infirmary also served as an infirmary for any civilians in the area who might need medical attention.

One Friday night, just after we had completed our supper, such as it was, we were told that there had been a serious automobile crash and the *chovshim* were to go to the infirmary at once. There we learned that a civilian van belonging to an Israeli company doing some work in Sinai had collided head on with a rental car full of tourists – and they were all being rushed to our infirmary. This was a terrible accident, and two of the people were already dead on arrival. Numerous others were injured, not all seriously, but one of the tourists, an American, was critically injured, with a ruptured spleen and other internal injuries. Thank goodness this time I was not alone, and there were some six to eight *chovshim* and *two* doctors available from whom we, the *chovshim*, were happy to take our orders. What four of us did was to force fluid into the critically wounded tourist's veins as fast as we could by standing on chairs around the examination table where he lay, holding the bags of fluid above our heads and squeezing the plastic bottles of IV fluid to get it to go in as fast as possible. Holding one's arms up for protracted periods is extremely tiring, and we thought ours would drop off. All this while we waited for an aircraft to land from Sharm el Sheik, the nearest major army base, to evacuate this man to hospital. It was touch-and-go, and the doctors were constantly monitoring whether his kidneys were still functioning. While we were attending to the American suddenly, from one moment to the next, our battalion doctor vanished into thin air. No one knew where he had gone. Absent for a few minutes, he then just as suddenly reappeared.

"Where did you go?" the other doctor asked.

"I went to get my dirty laundry. I reckoned that if I was going to have to fly to hospital in Tel Aviv with the wounded, at least I'd grab the opportunity to nip home and get my wife to do my laundry tonight!"

I was flabbergasted. How could a doctor be thinking about an opportunity to do his laundry at a time like this? After all, he was due to fly with two dead bodies, a critically injured man, and several other wounded, and all he could think of was his laundry. It was only many years later, when I became addicted to the television comedy M*A*S*H, that I understood that this was the kind of tragic event that served as the basis for the poignant humor of that wonderful series. I gradually learned to understand that if medical personnel did not distance themselves from the personal tragedy of the cases with which they dealt, they would not be able to carry on and function in the best possible way.

After what seemed like an eternity the plane arrived, and we evacuated the dead and wounded, subsequently learning that the American with the ruptured spleen had survived. Not being hardened doctors who live these traumas daily, this was exhilarating for us. And our doctor returned the following day with spanking clean underwear.

On another occasion, just as we were relaxing and preparing to go to sleep, we were told that we had to go out on a patrol. And, once again, yours truly was to be part of the patrol because of that never-ending need for the presence of a *chovesh*. We were not thrilled. We were told that two people had been stranded in the middle of Wadi

Piran, and that they needed to be 'rescued.' Wadi Piran is a dry river bed that runs from the Gulf into the heart of Sinai, to Saint Catherine's Monastery located at the foot of what is believed to be Mount Sinai, where Moses received the Ten Commandments. It is a good three hours' drive from where we were based, bouncing along over pebbles and rocks in this dry river bed, and it is wretchedly uncomfortable and hard on the back. When we finally found the people, it turned out that they were American tourists, a man and a woman, who had rented a Volkswagen Combi and were on their way to the monastery when they had broken down. Well, of course they had broken down: a Combi is a little camper/van, not a four-wheel drive, which sits very low on the road and is totally unsuited to driving through Sinai's wadis. They had broken an axle and were not going anywhere. They were petrified that they were going to be murdered during the night, and were extremely grateful to us for saving them. I regret to say that we were not that gracious in return. We took them back with us, and the following day sent a towing vehicle to get the Combi. A strange assignment for a *chovesh*.

Finally December 31, my wedding anniversary, arrived. This time it was my sixth. Still being very happily married (as I am today, thirty-eight years on), I was once again feeling utterly despondent, terribly sorry for myself, and not very cooperative. Just when I thought I had some free time after dark, someone came running into my room, all excited:

"Get ready! We're going on a patrol," he shouted.

"Not me again," I grumbled.

"Stop grumbling. You're very lucky that you are a *chovesh* and that you *have to* go. Many of the riflemen are vying for a place on this patrol."

"What's the attraction?" I asked unenthusiastically.

"We are going to pick up a sick Swedish female" (in Hebrew "Shvedit"), he cried excitedly.

Being in the army brings out all sorts of macho and sexist tendencies, and the prospect of being part of the group that was going to save a ravishing Swedish blonde in distress was nothing short of thrilling. To them, I might add, not to me, who was simply depressed about not being with my wife for our anniversary.

Once again we set off in the direction of St. Catherine's Monastery, looking for the vehicle we were supposed to meet up with, which was going to pass the sick Swede over for us to take back to the infirmary.

After many hours, we found the vehicle and asked where the Swedish girl was.

"What Swedish girl?" they asked. "There's no Swedish girl. It's a sick Bedouin woman."

She was having a gall bladder attack. Not too romantic.

"*Shvedit – Beduit*" had obviously sounded the same to the radio man – or maybe it was just wishful thinking.

The early seventies saw both growth and contraction in our family circle. My cousins from South Africa, Marie and Aaron, arrived in Israel, but my brother Steve and his wife Ami went the other way, returning to live in Johannesburg. The decision to leave Israel is not the kind of topic either easily or readily discussed, even among family members, in that country, and to this day we have never delved into their reasons for deciding to leave. One factor I know of in their decision was the recent death of Ami's father, leaving her mother alone in the world since Ami is an only child. However, as was the case with Jenny and me six years later, there was no doubt a myriad of factors impelling them towards their agonizing decision.

But there was growth in our immediate family, too: in April of 1971 our second daughter, Noa, was born in Jerusalem, and a few months later we moved from our Nili Street apartment to a larger one on Uziel Street in Bayit Vegan. Bayit Vegan is on the other side of the city from Nili Street, and in a somewhat less desirable area, which made it possible to buy a slightly larger place. Today, Bayit Vegan is a very religious neighborhood, and could I think be uncomfortable for non-observant Jews like ourselves. However, in the 1970s, although some of the roads in Bayit Vegan were religious, and one was even closed during the Sabbath, Uziel Street itself was a pleasant mixture of religious and secular. Jenny and I were both happy and proud of our little family and our new home. This apartment was even closer to where my parents lived than our previous one, something that was to become of increasing importance as my father's health declined.

The first half of 1973 went by fairly normally. Nationally the economy was doing well, the one cloud on the horizon being the occupation and the corrosive effect it was beginning to have on Israeli society. It was during this period that I began discussions with the authorities at the Hebrew University about the possibility of receiving a scholarship from them in order to go abroad in 1974 to do a Ph.D. in Applied Linguistics. My reasons for wanting to study abroad were the same as when I wanted to do my M.A.: the suitability of the program, together with the prospect of a scholarship that would enable me to devote myself to full time study without the distraction of having to earn a living. The plan was that Jenny would seek work as a librarian wherever I was studying in order to augment the income derived from the modest scholarship. By the end of the summer of 1973 I still did not have a definitive answer, but the indications were all positive. Jenny, for her part, had been working at the university library for several years, and had decided that she wanted to be a professional librarian. This meant that she needed to gain a graduate qualification in librarianship. Consequently we realized that if we were to go abroad for a few years in 1974, she needed to take this course in the preceding academic year, so as to be able to work as a professional librarian while I did my Ph.D. This was not going to be an easy time for her: by this stage, Lee was almost four and Noa two and a half. And, what is more, our financial circumstances required that Jenny work – at least part-time – so she was clearly destined to have a very, very busy year.

On the whole, though, a bright if crowded future. Yet it contained one shadow, spreading anxiety over our lives. This was the growing and inescapable awareness that something was clearly seriously wrong with my father. His speech had become more and more slurred, his movements were slow and ponderous, and he did not seem to be as alert as he should have been. After all, he was only sixty three years old.

And then came Yom Kippur 1973.

Part IV

THE YOM KIPPUR WAR

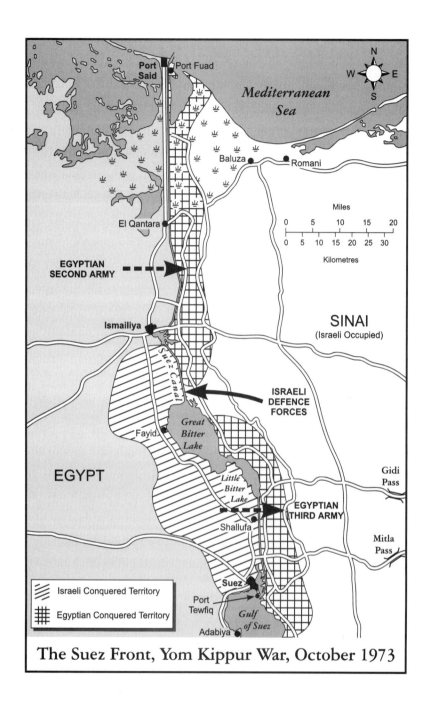

And then came Yom Kippur 1973.

Yom Kippur in Israel was always a strange day for non-religious people like Jenny and me, since we had both been brought up as non-observant but 'traditional' Jews; when I came to Israel, I abandoned the few traditions that I had observed in South Africa. I attribute this to two factors.

First, Israel in the 1960s and 1970s was an extremely polarized society religiously, leaving little room for people like us who wanted to observe and retain certain traditions, but were not willing to become any more religious than we were. There were no Progressive Jewish synagogues such as exist in North America – not Reform, Conservative or Reconstructionist – and I found myself becoming less and less observant and involved in anything religious. If one wanted to be involved, one needed to be more orthodox than we were interested in being, so instead I drifted further and further away from religious observance. The polarity between religious and secular Jews was just too sharp, and there was no middle ground – either you became more orthodox, or you became totally secular, and I chose the latter.

The second reason we moved away from synagogue attendance was that a major factor in our families' involvement in Jewish life and observances in South Africa had simply been as a form of identification with Jews. Obviously, when one is living in the Jewish state itself, there's no such need to identify.

In spite of where we stood religiously in those days, we nevertheless always respected the sanctity of Yom Kippur by not driving, and would walk about the streets marveling at the quiet and the calm. However, in all my years of living in Israel, I never spent Yom Kippur in the synagogue.

As it so happened, in 1973 my mother-in-law had come up from Tel Aviv to spend Yom Kippur with us, bringing with her a couple, Chloe and Aaron, who were visiting from South Africa. Aaron had grown up in Durban in the same apartment building as Jenny, and in South Africa the two families had been close, so it was delightful having them to stay, particularly as Jenny always derives such pleasure from meeting childhood friends. Neither of us had met Chloe before, but Aaron was just as warm, decent, frank and open as Jenny had remembered him, and I was glad to meet him and welcome him into our home.

On Kol Nidrei, the eve of Yom Kippur, we went outside to experience the quiet of a city normally resounding with the honking of horns and the constant throbbing of traffic. As we were standing outside our building, a chartered bus pulled up and a soldier jumped off and went into an adjacent building, but we thought nothing of it. The following morning, Aaron and I decided to take Lee and Noa for a walk before everyone got up. As we strolled around our neighborhood, I was surprised to notice quite a few cars moving – many more than I would have expected on Yom Kippur. Aaron had never been in Israel before so had nothing to compare this with, but I sensed that there was too much movement. And then, as we were passing a public building, a car screeched to a halt and a man got out and started putting up a sign on the fence. I knew that this was something military. "What's going on?" I asked him. All he would say over his shoulder was, "Listen to the BBC." (*Kol Yisrael*, Israel Radio, does not broadcast on Yom Kippur, which is why the man told me to listen to the BBC.) Being a reservist I realized that something serious must be happening, but did not immediately let on to Aaron what I suspected, although clearly there was some sort of major emergency. When I did tell Aaron, I suggested to him that we not say anything to any of the others so as not to alarm them. I said that I would call my *miluim* unit: if there was no answer, it would mean that all was well, but if someone answered, then it would mean that something big was afoot.

Without breathing a word to anyone else, I shut myself in our bedroom and called the number, but as many times as I tried the line it was always busy. I now knew beyond a shadow of a doubt that this was serious. Aaron and I decided not to say anything yet, but to wait for the BBC news as the man in the car had recommended. I, for my part, sensing that a call up was imminent, quietly packed a bag of underwear, toiletries and the like ready for the inevitable summons.

At 2.00 p.m. I insisted that we listen to the BBC, although Jenny could not understand why I was so persistent. Even as we were learning that Egypt had attacked Israel at the Suez Canal and that Egyptian soldiers were streaming across the canal, with Syria concurrently attacking from the north, the air raid sirens went off and we all rushed to the shelter.

Our apartment was directly opposite a large synagogue, and no sooner had the sirens begun their eerie wailing than people started pouring out. In fact, for some years after this, our daughters associated air raid sirens with synagogues! There was pandemonium in the shelter, which was in the basement of the building, and in true Israeli fashion there were more opinions being voiced and more commentaries on events than people in the shelter. No one was actually saying it, but we all realized that the situation was serious. None of us knew at that point just how serious the situation was, and that *Tzahal* was to be put to the toughest test in its history.

We spent some time in the shelter, and then the all clear sounded. This was not like the Six Day War in Jerusalem – this time the city was never bombed, and to the best of my knowledge the civilians were not sent back to the shelters again throughout the entire war. In my case, for reasons I shall make apparent, I was not to remain in Jerusalem for very much longer.

No sooner had the all clear sounded than my parents arrived with all their perishable food, saying that they wanted to be with us rather than be alone. The tables had turned in six short years, and whereas Jenny had leaned on them and relied on them so much for help and support and love in 1967, this time it was they who were in serious need of our support. But, despite our good intentions, history decreed otherwise, and in the event it proved to be not *we* who provided that support, but Jenny *alone*.

Minutes later another South African from Durban, Sue, arrived. She was our closest friend, and had bought an apartment close to us. She was single and not in the best of health, and did not have any family whatsoever in Israel, so we had become her family and she would move in with us to recuperate after her numerous stays in hospital. We were now 10 people in all in our modest two-bedroom apartment: my parents, the four of us, my mother-in-law, Sue, and Aaron and Chloe.

Having Aaron and Chloe, tourists, with us at this critical and desperate time was strange, to say the least. Everyone except for Chloe remained calm and controlled. All she wanted to do was to go home to her children in South Africa. No one could blame her – this was not her war, or her country, and she was petrified. Aaron is what one would describe in Yiddish as a *gutte* – a good soul, and no sooner had the sirens begun their hideous wail than he turned to Chloe and said, "I think I should sign up with the army to help."

"You'll do no such thing," Chloe retorted. "We're getting out of Israel as soon as we can, and we're never coming back!"

To be fair to them, they had been due to fly out that very night, and the plan had been that my mother–in-law would take them to the airport after Yom Kippur ended. Of course that never happened, as the airport was closed and no flights arrived or left until the situation had settled somewhat. Chloe's palpable anxiety and fear did not make her popular that day. Of course she was deeply worried and frightened, but she was unable to appreciate what the rest of the people she was with, indeed the whole country, were going through at that moment.

As soon as we were allowed out of the shelter, Chloe said to me that she had to speak to her mother in South Africa to alert her about what was going on and warn her that they would not be arriving on the flight they had booked. Now international phoning was not very sophisticated in Israel in those days, and in any case the lines would be jammed with people making contact with family elsewhere in the country and abroad. I said that I would try and get through for her. There was no direct dialing – it was all through the operator, assuming you could get through to the switchboard at all. I settled down at the phone, and after about twenty minutes of trying, miraculously I got through to her mother in Johannesburg and passed Chloe the receiver.

Chloe was clearly anxious not to alarm her mother. While I could not hear what her mother was saying, of course, I could guess from Chloe's responses, and this is what I heard her say:

"Mum, there's a little problem on the border, and we're not going to be able to get home tomorrow as planned." PAUSE

"I understand, Mum, but you see the airport is closed at present." PAUSE

"I realize that this is putting you out, but what can I do?" PAUSE

"But Mum, you don't understand. No planes are leaving Israel at present. There's fighting on the border." PAUSE

"I *understand* that you've invited a whole lot of people to welcome us back, but what can we do?" PAUSE

"I'm sorry, but you'll have to call and cancel. I'm really sorry." PAUSE

"I know you've gone to a lot of trouble planning this little party, and I'm sorry."

It ultimately took Chloe and Aaron several days before they could get a flight out of Israel, and to the best of my knowledge, true to her word, they have never been back. If truth be told, the interaction between Chloe and her mother provided the rest of us with some welcome light relief.

The numbers sheltering in the apartment were to drop from ten to nine within the hour. My call up came very soon after the all clear sounded, and I left on that fateful day of October 6, to return as a discharged soldier the following March. As I think back on it, the parting from Jenny, the girls and the rest of the family was strange – no tears or hysterics – just a lot of hugging and kissing. Jenny (like my mother) is an eternal optimist, and I believe that this helped her through all these scary times. It was certainly her courage and her positive approach that made it all bearable for me. As for my parents, I believe that my mother was not so much an optimist as an excellent actor.

That night of October 6 was a very strange one. I spent it mustering soldiers from my unit, and this necessitated traveling throughout the night on the bus that I had been allocated to several different points in the country collecting other reservists. Whomever we approached, even when we had woken them from a deep sleep, received us with words of encouragement and food and hot drinks. That was an eerie and unreal night, but it provided me with further evidence of Israel's unique character: here we were, gathering up families' loved ones to go off and fight in a desperate war of survival, and yet we were received warmly and with love. We felt appreciated, and were keenly aware that there was a strong sense that we were doing this for our families and others – a sense that had been imbued in me by Dudu in his speeches before the outbreak of the Six Day War. Israel was seriously threatened at that moment, all our lives were in danger, and people truly appreciated us.

We brought all the people we had gathered in the bus back to our unit's assembly point in Jerusalem. And so began my five months and one week in *Tzahal* in the Yom Kippur War – which was to prove a vastly different experience from the Six Day War. Every soldier has his own experiences in a war. In some ways, for me, the Yom Kippur War was not nearly so bad as 1967, but in other ways it was much worse. One thing is certain – it was totally different: the dangers were different, the duration was different, the location was different, and the mood was certainly different. At no time did we ever feel any excitement, any thrill of euphoria, even when the tide finally turned in Israel's favor.

Until that fateful day of October 6 the Israeli and Egyptian armies had been dug in, in fortified *mutzavim* opposite each other on the two sides of the Suez Canal. On the morning after Yom Kippur, when war broke out, and before being sent to guard the Jordanian border to the east, I was in an army base wondering and worrying about friends and acquaintances who I knew were in *miluim* and who had been stationed along the Canal. I knew that they included Dov, an acquaintance from South Africa, and Uri, both colleagues from the university. It turned out that Dov had been doing his regular *miluim* in a *mutzav* right on the Suez Canal when the Egyptians attacked. This was to have been a period of *miluim* not that different from the *miluim* I described on the Jordan River. The only difference was that the 'line' along the Canal was even quieter than the Jordanian front at that particular time. The army had sent as many soldiers as they felt they could spare home from the front to be with their families for Yom Kippur. Not Dov. He was there, in the *mutzav*, when the Egyptians attacked, and his mutzav was quickly overrun. Soon after this, Dov was declared missing in action, and subsequently declared dead by the Army Rabbinate. His body was never found.

I was also deeply worried about Uri. He and I had chatted at the university a few weeks earlier and he had told me that he was off to *miluim* on the Canal. All of a sudden, at the assembly point in Jerusalem, I saw Uri walking towards me. I ran to him and hugged him: "How wonderful to see you – I thought you were down at the Suez Canal."

"Can you believe it?" said Uri, "My unit *is* at the Canal, but I was home on leave for Yom Kippur!" The timing of that leave saved Uri's life, but many of his friends and comrades disappeared in those first few days, never to be found.

Some time after being discharged I was doing some recordings of language lessons, when the sound technician told me a remarkable story: He, too, had been in a *mutzav* on the Canal, and not on leave, when the war began and the Egyptians had attacked. Because it was supposed to be quiet and even boring in *miluim* on the Canal, he had taken his portable professional tape recorder with him, "in case there was anything interesting to record." The moment the war started he began narrating what he could see and hear, and recording exchanges between the different people in his *mutzav*. He was one of the lucky ones who managed to retreat from his *mutzav* unhurt, and ultimately he made a radio documentary with the recordings he had. This was a remarkable program, and Jenny and I were deeply moved when we heard it. He was lucky to have been able to get away because his *mutzav*, like Dov's, was overrun by the Egyptians.

At the same time as the Egyptians hurled themselves across the Canal, the Syrians attacked from the north-east, forcing Israel to fight on two fronts at the same time. Moreover, there was a serious danger that King Hussein of Jordan would attack from the east. After all, he had done so in 1967, and had lost a substantial amount of his territory to Israel, territory that he might now have reasonably felt he had a chance of regaining were he to throw in his lot with the Syrians and Egyptians. My unit was sent for a couple of weeks to the Jordanian border, to the Jordan Valley a little north of Jericho, to guard against the opening of a third front. I found myself not that far from where I had served in a *mutzav* a few years earlier.

As it happened, the period my unit spent on the Jordanian border lasted for a couple of weeks, but turned out to be militarily uneventful, albeit somewhat incongruous at the same time. We knew that Israel was fighting for its life as it had never had to fight before; we knew that Israeli positions had been overrun near the Suez Canal and up near the Golan Heights; we knew that many prisoners had been taken and others were missing in action; we knew that there were very heavy losses; and we knew that Jordan could attack at any moment. But the Jordanian border mercifully remained completely quiet – King Hussein never attacked.

Coupled with all the terrible news that we were receiving – from the Egyptian front in particular – came other, more hopeful tidings. Ariel Sharon had led a force westwards across the Suez Canal and taken control of a narrow 'sausage' of land on the west side – the African side – of the Canal. Israel up till then had never taken control of any territory on the western side of the Canal, on the continent of Africa. Sharon's was a daring military feat, and one that in many ways turned the tide of that war, because Israel now had a very important bargaining chip: a piece of land stretching from half way into the city of Suez in the south to the outskirts of the city of Ismailia in the north. Even more important in many ways, this feat of Sharon's resulted in the Egyptian Third Army, which was occupying a piece of land on 'our' side (the east side) of the Canal, becoming completely surrounded by Israeli forces, and cut off from its supply lines. It was to fall to U.S. Secretary of State Henry Kissinger to try to disentangle the mess in which the two sides found themselves once the most vicious fighting had died down. And it was here that the term 'shuttle diplomacy' was popularized. This 'disengagement,' as it came to be called, was to take a long time, and in its own way to have a direct impact on my life.

So this, then, was the military situation: a desperate battle was being fought against the Egyptians in the south and the Syrians in the north-east, and here we were, a combat unit that had fought in one of the most critical battles of the Six Day War, stationed on the Jordanian border, doing nothing more than standing guard in case Jordan attacked. And Jordan did not attack – that border remained totally quiet for the entire time that we were stationed there and, indeed, throughout the war. Ironically for my unit, it was at this point as quiet and as uneventful as the quietest period of *miluim* I had ever done on the border, except of course for the terrible news flowing in from the other fronts. News of deaths and injuries were coming through daily, and everyone waited with baited breath for each broadcast for the names of the fallen. But all we did was to do guard duty as if there was nothing untoward going on.

Early October is generally still hot in Israel, and it was certainly extremely hot where we were in the Jordan Valley, below sea level, near Jericho. The hardest thing we had to do during that two-week period was to keep cool and to avoid dehydration. As medics, our main task was to ensure that all the soldiers in our unit drank enough. As *chovshim* in the *ta'agad*, we were required to go around from platoon to platoon holding 'drinking parades.' These were not at all what they might sound like. What we would do was to have all the soldiers line up in threes, and in our presence they were required to drink at least one full canteen of water each. *Tzahal*, over the years, had done extensive research into the question of the relationship between functioning well and drinking enough, and had come up with definitive data proving that the more water soldiers drank, the better they functioned – a far cry from the prevailing wisdom when I was in basic training. But this raised a logistical question: how do you get soldiers to drink in the blazing hot desert, for example, when all the water becomes lukewarm or even warmer, and often is quite foul tasting. Some simple but no less ingenious solutions were found. Units were supplied with water tankers that could be pulled behind a jeep or command car, but these became really warm as they stood in the baking sun. So a device was made, which worked as follows: each unit was supplied with what looked like a normal civilian insulated picnic box, together with blocks of ice taking up the full space of the picnic box. The picnic box was attached to the water tanker. Water pipes ran up and down through the insulation of the box and exited with a tap on the other side. As the warm water from the tanker ran through the pipes in the walls of the picnic box, it became really cold and inviting to drink. And the blocks of ice in their insulated boxes took such a long time to melt that the soldiers had cold water for hours and hours. Moreover, they were supplied with some fruit flavoring similar in taste to Kool Aid, which was available in powdered form next to the water box to make the water more palatable.

Our *ta'agad* team was a disparate one. Our doctor was a highly trained specialist in internal medicine, and the group of medics came from all over the globe, with very different backgrounds and interests. But we managed to get along pretty well most of the time. As rank in

Tzahal, and particularly in *miluim*, is not of great significance, none of us wore our stripes, but all the medics were either corporals or sergeants – and it made absolutely no difference anyway. In addition to the medics and doctor, there was an ambulance driver and a radio man. For some reason our *ta'agad's* regular radio man was not with us for the Yom Kippur War, and a new man, Tuviya, was sent to us. Tuviya, it turned out, was the younger brother of a colleague of mine at the Hebrew University High School, and this immediately gave us something in common. But we did not need that connection, as we became firm friends, maintained and enlarged our friendship back in civilian life to include Jenny and his wife Sarah, and I'm happy to say that it flourishes to this day. When we went to Edinburgh in 1974 for three years for graduate study, it was Tuviya who managed our financial affairs, including supervising the tenants in our sublet apartment.

To be completely honest, that two-week period was deadly boring. It almost sounds blasphemous to use that sort of terminology when Israel was fighting for its very existence, but it is true. And speaking completely selfishly, I was not complaining. As a *chovesh* in the *ta'agad*, we were responsible for the health of the soldiers from the different companies and platoons in our battalion, and this included illness in addition to injury of which, thankfully, there was none. On one particular day, I was instructed to travel in the ambulance to the fully equipped infirmary in Jericho with a soldier who had been brought to us running a high fever. While there, I was also to pick up some supplies. I was quite delighted, as this "outing" would fill the best part of the day. What is more, I would be able to pick up the mail, go to the army cafeteria and get a cold drink and a snack, and maybe even call Jenny, with whom I'd been unable to speak since the call up.

To my delight, I discovered that at the place where the infirmary was, out in the open, the army had constructed a sort of doorless telephone booth so soldiers could call home – free. There was absolutely no privacy, of course, so inevitably anyone waiting their turn to call could not avoid hearing every word of your conversation. Mind you, even if the booth had had doors no one would have closed them; it was stiflingly hot merely standing in the sun waiting to call, so telephoning from a closed booth would have been unbearable.

But as with so many things in the army, there was a catch – in fact there were *two* catches. The first was that this was a military line, monitored for such security breaches as divulging one's location, and the second was that every unit in the area knew about this one measly telephone, and the line that day was close to a hundred soldiers long. But I had no other plans, and as the ambulance driver also wanted to call home we decided to join the line. When I said to him that this would mean that we would be away rather a long time, he said, "Nonsense. I do this every time I am here, so they won't expect us any earlier than I usually get back." We waited and waited for our turn, chatting and joking with the people around us, and making editorial comments on some of the things we heard the soldier on the telephone saying.

When we were about six or seven men away from the front of the line, we heard the following conversation between a soldier and, we presumed, his wife:

"Hi, *motek* (sweetie). How are you?" PAUSE

"I'm fine. How are the kids?" PAUSE

"What's new?" PAUSE

"I cannot tell you where I am stationed." PAUSE

"But I'm not allowed to tell." PAUSE

"Don't you understand. It's against military regulations." PAUSE

"No, I'm *not* going to tell you. I will get into trouble." PAUSE

"Okay. Let me think a minute." PAUSE

By this stage we were getting both quite involved in and quite irritated by what was going on. Here we were, sweltering, dying to have our turn, and this fellow's stupid wife would not let go – she absolutely insisted on him breaking an army regulation and telling her where he was.

"Just a minute, I'm thinking how to put this." PAUSE

Suddenly his face lit up.

"I'm not allowed to say where I am, but it's the place where Joshua made the walls fall down by blowing his trumpets."

About 10 of us burst out laughing and began applauding. Military secrecy had been kept intact and remained inviolate.

I finally got my turn and was able to talk to Jenny and tell her that I was fine and safe, but the conversation was dominated by her telling me of the deaths of those friends and family of which she was already aware. There was Gideon, the younger brother of Adam, Nadav's best friend, whom I mentioned earlier, the sons of two of Jenny's distant cousins and, she told me, she had heard that a substantial number of graduates whom I had taught at the Hebrew University High School had been killed, but she did not have details. Sadly, this was the pattern of such conversations at this time. This was not a six-day wonder war with limited casualties. And the talk everywhere was about people we each knew who had been killed. The mood was indeed somber.

Israel is such a remarkable country in so many ways, and one is the way in which the mood of the moment is captured in song. As I have described, the Six Day War generated so many songs – funny, cheeky, and poignant. The Yom Kippur War, on the other hand, yielded really only one truly memorable song, again written by Naomi Shemer – it is called *Lu Yehi – Let It Be*. The words truly capture the mood of the time – somber, trying to be optimistic, and praying for the strength and safety of all our loved ones. Even now, as I write these words decades later, my eyes are full of tears and there is a lump in my throat.

After about two weeks on the Jordanian border, we were told that we were being moved. Soldiers do not take kindly to being moved – somehow you bond with the place you are stationed, however awful it may be, and you always fear that the new place will prove to be even worse. Rumors flew as to where we were being sent – there had been bitter fighting on the Syrian as well as the Egyptian borders, and I don't know which direction aroused less enthusiasm among us: going north or going south. The situation on both borders was calming down, although the intertwining of the Egyptian and Israeli forces in their respective newly captured enclaves, with no clear-cut borders, made the Suez front situation highly volatile and complicated. Mind you, it didn't really matter what *we* thought or wanted, because we knew that we were about to be told that we would be going somewhere – and that that was an order and the end of the matter.

As far as I could discern, the decision about where we were being sent was changed several times. But then we could not always distinguish between rumors and facts, and the former were abundant and contradictory. What we knew for certain was that we were moving. We were told to pack up everything and to stand to at the ready. One of the major disadvantages of being a *ta'agad* medic was the vast amount of equipment that the *ta'agad* had, all of which had to be packed and loaded whenever we moved. After all, the *ta'agad* included several large tents, and vast containers of medical supplies which were crushingly heavy. To pack up for a major move took several hours. Our *ta'agad* alone had a huge truck full of equipment, an ambulance, plus personnel: a doctor, a radio man and the seven or eight medics along with our own personal side arms and equipment, the last of which was itself not insignificant.

By early evening we and the rest of the battalion, with all its light and heavy equipment, including things like field kitchens, sand bags, and much, much more, were ready. The logistics of moving a large group of soldiers with all their equipment in a long, motley convoy of vehicles was anything but simple, and there was a definite air of hectic and fevered expectancy as our officers rushed around barking orders, planning the order of departure of the vehicles, and determining the distance apart they should travel so that they were close to each other but not sitting targets for air attacks. It must have been around 7:00 p.m. before we finally set out, still not knowing if we were going north to Syria or south to Egypt.

In the end we were informed that we were crossing the Suez Canal, to hold the northern end of the enclave of land that Sharon's expeditionary force had captured in the early days of the fighting. This meant that we would be crossing westwards over to the Egyptian side of the Suez Canal, in other words crossing onto the African continent, then wheeling right (northwards) in the direction of Ismailia – not that I had *any* idea of the map or the terrain at that point. Jokes began to fly from that moment on that, for some of us, we were 'going home' – after all, many of us were from Africa: Tunisia, Morocco, Libya, Algeria, and South Africa.

The journey down to the Canal was in itself an experience. Our battalion was loaded onto a long convoy of vehicles of every possible description: military transports like armored troop carriers, jeeps, and command cars, as well as civilian vehicles such as buses, trucks large and small, and vans of different shapes and sizes which had been temporarily requisitioned by *Tzahal*. The *ta'agad* team, for example, had a panel van that had been fitted with stretchers so as to serve as an ambulance, but little did we know that, once we crossed the Canal, such a vehicle would be useless in the soft sand of the unpaved roads, and would bog down almost immediately. While time remains something of a blur to me, I do know for certain that our advance to the Suez front lasted longer than overnight. Not only did we travel slowly, but there seemed to be an interminable number of stops along the way. Sleeping in that van was a challenge. There were at least five of us plus a huge amount of personal equipment, and to this day I wonder how we all managed to fit in, let alone sleep. At that time, with all the wildly varying experiences I'd had in *Tzahal*, I used to joke that I was going to write a book called *Places I Have Slept*, and that civilian van *en route* to Suez would definitely have featured.

Although the trip was long and uncomfortable, it was almost fun – rather like setting out on some bizarre kind of adventure. We seemed to stop a lot, and we had numerous opportunities to buy sandwiches or humus in pita and the like from roadside kiosks along the way. I remember stopping during the night somewhere in the Ashkelon area, I think, and discovering that we were at a major intersection of two interurban roads. We were allowed to get out to stretch our legs, and there at the corner was a prostitute trying to pick up clients from passing cars. Well, you can easily imagine what a hard time a group of bored soldiers gave her, asking her lots of silly questions and proffering many heavily humorous suggestions, such as whether or not she'd be prepared to open a branch office near the Canal. If she had been a shy, retiring young woman, she would have been uncomfortable and would, no doubt, have run as fast as she could in the opposite direction. However, being the woman of the world that she was, she gave back as fast and as sharply as she received and we, and she, ended by sharing a really good laugh.

Eventually, the following day, we reached the Suez Canal, or at least we came close to it. It was not much more than a week since Sharon's force had captured this territory across the Canal, and there was still serious danger from Egyptian snipers and commando units. The Israeli expeditionary force on the west side was dangerously vulnerable at that time, and there was always the fear that there would be a counterattack by the Egyptians that could cut them off, as Sharon's force had done to the Egyptian Third Army on the eastern bank of the canal. This was to lead to the building of a road across the Canal by *Tzahal* in order to secure our supply lines of communication and enable us to conduct an orderly and strategic withdrawal should circumstances necessitate it.

As we moved closer to the Canal, we encountered a number of Israeli units dug in to defend this important but vulnerable crossing point, the only one at which you could cross the Canal, making it strategically of great significance. Our convoy had halted a few kilometers before the Canal – we could not see it from where we were – and given the extreme danger, we were sent through one vehicle at a time, only proceeding when given the word by the units responsible for guarding the crossing point.

The Suez Canal may not be particularly wide, but it is still striking suddenly to come across this perfectly straight ribbon of blue water in the middle of the never-ending desert sand. Jenny and I had taken one trip through Sinai shortly after the Six Day War, but we had never been to the Canal, and to see this waterway – a real engineering feat of the nineteenth century, a wonder of the world – was truly exciting. The fact that *Tzahal* had secured a foothold on its western bank was extremely important in determining the outcome of the war on the Egyptian front.

At this stage, the crossing was done on temporary pontoon bridges that had been assembled by the Engineering Corps. These were far from sturdy constructions, and imparted the sensation of bouncing as you crossed on them. Being as narrow as it is, crossing the Canal took little time, but I couldn't help but be aware that we were engaged in doing something historic, and was appropriately anxious to mark the occasion in some suitable way. But I had no idea what to do.

When the Suez Canal was being built, parallel to it and about a mile or two to the west, a second canal was built, called the Sweetwater Canal. This canal was built to provide drinking water for the men building the Suez Canal, and subsequently to irrigate the land between the two canals. As a result, this strip of land, a narrow ribbon of lush green set in an apparently limitless expanse of sandy desert, is indeed intensely cultivated with orange groves, the fruits of which we were to enjoy a few months later when they ripened. However to call this "Sweetwater" was a comic misnomer – the water is infested with bilharzia, and many of the local population in the area suffer from it. Bilharzia is a horrible disease contracted from parasitic worms that live in tropical, stagnant water, and that can enter the body through the pores of the skin, settling and multiplying in the veins that carry blood from the intestines to the liver, causing all sorts of organ malfunction. Bilharzia notwithstanding, this narrow belt blossomed with profuse vegetation and trees, and yielded abundant harvests of fruit, particularly citrus, unlike the classic sand dune desert wasteland through which we had just traveled.

After we had crossed the Suez Canal, we turned northwards between the two canals, and began making our way towards Ismailia. The excitement of the crossing quickly evaporated. A dismal sight met our eyes, and one that I hate to remember – never-ending lines of

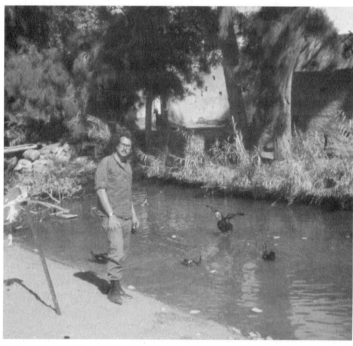

At the Sweetwater Canal, October, 1973.

poor, barefooted Egyptian peasants from the area streaming northwards towards Ismailia with whatever of their worldly goods they could carry or load onto their donkeys. They were heading to safety because of *me* – because of this invading force – and I was the invader. This was harsh reality, and I was horrified by my role in this human misery, one I truly hated, and my heart went out to these people who were turning into refugees right before my eyes. These simple rural folk knew that the Israeli soldiers were coming into their villages in ever greater numbers, and understandably they panicked, not knowing that we would not do either them or their property any harm. Nevertheless they made the classic decision that people in such a plight have always made throughout the ages: they packed up what they could and headed away from their enemy, in this case to Ismailia, which lay beyond the most northerly point to which *Tzahal* advanced. I am happy to say that those of the local population who stayed indeed came to no harm while we occupied their territory. But actually witnessing a line of refugees fleeing to sanctuary from me and what I represented was infinitely saddening.

The area we traveled through or, more accurately, often had to push our ambulance through, was cultivated but at the same time extremely poor. The villages often had only one or two stone or concrete buildings: a mosque, and sometimes the local administration building. All the other buildings were mud huts with mud floors and no running water or electricity. We were soon to learn that the most common creature in that area is the flea. In the first few nights we were there we were wakened by them hopping all over us, and we medics were inundated with requests for something to keep them away and also to treat flea bites. The Medical Corps did what they could and supplied what they could, but the only thing that really helped was our own bodies' developing a resistance to these critters. Within a few weeks we became totally unaffected by them, and were seldom bitten. But whenever a new soldier joined us, it was the same story all over again.

Where our battalion actually ended up was right on the outskirts of the Egyptian city of Ismailia, with the Egyptian army dug in some 150 meters away. Our platoons were deployed along the improvised front line, which ran through the fields of the peasants. Headquarters

Company, to which the *ta'agad* belonged, was eventually moved about a kilometer back into the stone administration building in one of the villages. This was a tiny and extremely poor village, and virtually all the villagers had fled northwards so that we encountered very few of the local population.

The only other stone building in the village was the mosque. From the minaret, you could see not far away the outlines of buildings on the outskirts of Ismailia, but *Tzahal* never entered the city. The other landmark in the area that we could see when we went on patrols, just north of our line, was the Memorial to the Unknown Soldier at Jebel Mariam, erected by the British in memory of the fallen of World War I.

Everyone, including the military authorities, was much taken with the fact that we had crossed to a different continent, thereby qualifying us to write "Africa" on postcards and letters home. We were in Africa for four and a half never-ending months, and there was little that we experienced in that period that was dramatic, fun, noteworthy, heroic or enjoyable. In fact, I hated every minute of the time we were there, but like everyone else had no choice in the matter. Israel was at war, and all had to play their parts in protecting the country. If I did not do mine, whom could I expect to protect my family and my home?

It was really quite unbelievable. We had arrived in Africa, were there to hold a strategically vital piece of recently captured land, and we were to dig in a few meters from the Egyptian soldiers. And what is even more unbelievable is that in the first weeks we were there we had no fortified positions, no trenches, not even any sandbagged positions. The only thing that separated us from the Egyptian soldiers was a piece of white plastic marking tape lying on the ground – the kind of tape you might use to mark out a temporary soccer field in a park. We were so close to the Egyptians that in the quiet of night, while guarding, we could hear them talking – we could even hear the noise of a match being struck. It is hardly surprising that the line was tense and that there was shooting in one or both directions almost every night. Both sides were jittery. We knew how close they were to us, they knew how close we were to them, and we were both aware of our vulnerability. As a result, soldiers on both sides did not hesitate to open fire at anything they thought looked or sounded suspicious. But what did this mean?

Even if it is a short burst of light arms fire that goes off while you are guarding and it hits no one, the natural and correct thing is to fire back. This is bound to evoke a further response, and before you know where you are, there's a furious exchange of small arms fire; sometimes this even led to calling up artillery support, at which point things began escalating rapidly. Sniping was another serious danger – to both sides. Snipers would fire at our soldiers whenever they got them in their sights, and we lost one member of our battalion that way, and always had to be careful never to expose ourselves as targets in their telescopic sights. Unlike the British tradition of burying a soldier where he falls, Israel makes every effort to retrieve the body and then to arrange burial at the military cemetery nearest to the deceased's place of residence. In fact, this policy of always trying to retrieve a body has been the subject of some debate in Israel, because it sets the time honored principle in Judaism of 'respect for the dead' against the not uncommon reality of other soldiers endangering, and in some case losing, their lives to retrieve the body of a comrade.

There was also the problem of infiltration by Egyptian commando units, and this happened several times in the area where I was stationed. In fact, on one occasion, I had to treat a captured wounded commando infiltrator, my first experience of treating an enemy soldier, and I took particular care to give him the same attention that one of our own soldiers would have received. I carried out all the procedures that were required of me, but attending to the wounds of "the enemy" was a new and somehow awkward experience.

After a few days of being right on the front line, Headquarters Company including the *ta'agad* was moved about a kilometer back, and found itself on the ground floor of a now deserted two storey stone building that had been the offices of the regional government in the area. We quickly settled in and became accustomed to our new surroundings and to a war that was now static – there was no movement of troops on either side of the line, and what we were required to do was simply to hold the line.

As *chovshim*, we were also responsible for the general heath of the battalion, both in terms of illness and of injury. This meant that, when things were quiet militarily, we used to travel around in the ambulance from platoon to platoon checking that everyone was well, that basic hygiene was being observed as far as was possible, and treating any soldier who was unwell but not ill enough to necessitate moving him to the *ta'agad* or to a field hospital. I should point out that the army had by then realized that the van we were using as an ambulance was useless in these conditions, and had replaced it with a proper four-wheel-drive military ambulance.

I quite enjoyed these patrols and visits to the other platoons, since they helped to pass the time and afforded me the opportunity to visit my many friends in the different units. We were invariably hospitably received, and there was always someone around to chat to since time lay heavy on everyone's hands. I was also thoroughly intrigued to see and taste what the different groups were doing with their military rations in order to try to make the food palatable. Being small groups, they were really quite inventive, and they did much better gastronomically than we did in Headquarters Company, where inedible food was prepared for a large group by army cooks. We always tried to plan to reach one of the smaller units with a good reputation for cooking just as they were serving lunch.

On the many days that we did not go out on a visit to the platoons, we were required to do two hours of guard duty during daylight hours, but apart from that had few daytime duties. In such circumstances it is hardly surprising that we developed the ability to sleep for many, many hours in an effort to pass the time. We were also required to stand guard duty every night for four hours, which may partially explain why we spent so much of the day asleep, since guard duty was invariably tense and frequently quite scary, and on numerous occasions I came under fire. However the Egyptians, like us, were simply blazing away in the dark, and I emerged unscathed.

In the midst of all this tedium and fear, humor managed a brief intrusion when 'flu began to spread among the Israeli soldiers. It was winter, and although it was quite warm during the day – we walked around in light sweaters – it became bitterly cold at night, and several soldiers fell sick. We were given orders by the Brigade doctor that we were to give each and every soldier in the battalion a flu shot – no small undertaking. The routine we followed was to radio ahead to a unit informing them that we were on the way, and asking the officers to have the soldiers lying one next to the other, face down, bums at the ready, prepared to receive the shot. Then we arrived on the scene and, rather like the production line in Charlie Chaplin's *Modern Times*, made our way along the rows injecting one bum after another. In retrospect, I wish I had photographed this delightful scene.

There were, however, odd occasions on which the exchanges of fire became more serious, and heavier weaponry was used by both sides. On one occasion, a serious incident began a few minutes after I had returned from leave in Jerusalem. My mother and Jenny always made sure that I was well equipped with 'goodies' of all sorts when I returned. On that day, before I'd even had time to stow my backpack with my goodies and clean laundry the shooting began. We all grabbed our helmets and rushed to our positions. Bullets were flying in all directions. And then I felt like a snack. I opened my backpack, took out a large slab of chocolate, and began offering it to the soldiers stationed nearest to me, one of whom became incensed: "How can you eat chocolate in the middle of a serious incident?" he asked.

"Why not?" I replied.

"We might be killed at any moment," was his answer.

"All the more reason to eat it now," I said with a smile.

He was not amused, and the conversation ended right there.

The most serious incident occurred while I was away on leave in Jerusalem. When I left, everything was normal, with life going along in its usual humdrum way, day following day, with little out of the ordinary ever occurring. But while I was away an exchange of fire right along the line flared up, and in no time the Egyptians were firing Katyusha rockets as well as mortar shells and other types of artillery. An ex-American, Meir, in one of our platoons was seriously injured. He was standing in a firing pit that was about five and a half feet deep so that you could look out, rest your arms on the ground and fire from there. Meir was hit by shrapnel from a Katyusha – one arm was blown right off, and he also suffered severe damage to his face, losing half of his nose. He was bleeding profusely from the arteries in his arm as the soldiers in his unit rushed him by jeep to the *ta'agad* where, only thanks to the brilliant medical skills of our battalion doctor, Shlomo, was his life saved.

The Egyptians must have known (or assumed) that we would have a defensive position in the only stone building in the area – the one whose ground floor was being used as the *ta'agad* – because the building suffered a direct hit from a Katyusha rocket, totally destroying the upper floor. Some of the soldiers from Headquarters Company had been sleeping up there, and two of them were killed instantly. The *ta'agad* team slept on the ground floor, so none of our group was hurt in this attack. A truck full of equipment went up in flames, and there was other damage, too, but not to our major medical equipment on the ground floor. This was a serious incident, with the deaths, injuries and destruction, and our men were badly shaken. I came back from leave to a very different scene from the one I had left. Our base was now a severely damaged one-story building, a distinctly chilling reminder that there could never be any room for complacency.

There were some strange aspects to the African campaign that seemed to belong only in the pages of story books. One day, while I was visiting one of the platoons right at the front, all of a sudden we saw something pale blue moving in the tall grass; it seemed to be coming towards us. We bristled, ready for any eventuality. Rifles at the ready, we were suddenly confronted by a group of about eight to ten United Nations soldiers – peacekeepers – walking towards us, carrying their pale blue flag and wearing matching helmets. They were on a peacekeeping foot patrol between the Israeli and Egyptian lines, and had come to say hello. They were Scandinavian and spoke excellent English, and we had a pleasant conversation with them before they moved on. They, too, seemed deeply bored with what they were doing, although to my eyes, in the last third of the twentieth century, with all the awesome fire power assembled by both sides, it amazed me to have come upon these unarmed peacekeepers walking through the brush between the two hostile armies.

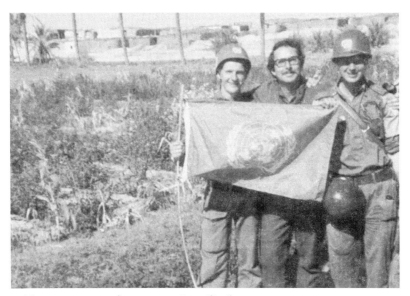

With two U.N. peacekeepers near Ismailia, late 1973.

Another strange event, unheard of in those days, was the meeting between our battalion commander and the Egyptian commander in the area. It was early 1974 and, to the best of my knowledge, there had been *no* direct talks between Israel and any of its Arab neighbors. When we heard that thanks to the efforts of Henry Kissinger, who was trying to broker an end to the fighting and a troop disengagement, there was going to be this meeting under the supervision of the United Nations commander in the area, we were dumbfounded. Needless to say, at our level no details of any kind were furnished about the discussions themselves, but we were explicitly told one thing: at this meeting both commanders complained that the other side's soldiers on guard duty were too quick to open fire, and that this was causing an unnecessary escalation in tension and injuries. Both commanders agreed that part of the problem was that the guards were all so tense. So an agreement was struck, what I have come to call 'the twenty second rule.' It was agreed that when there was a burst of fire from one side, the other side would wait twenty seconds before returning the fire, and if nothing further transpired in those twenty seconds, they would not fire back. This peculiar rule, which sounds more like one used to regulate a sporting contest rather than for application to soldiers on active duty was, nevertheless, strictly adhered to, and on numerous occasions of which I'm aware an incident was averted by applying it. Both sides scrupulously observed it, and the situation at night immediately became much calmer.

At some point close to the actual troop disengagement date, some of our soldiers went down to the line and spoke to Egyptian soldiers and exchanged Israeli for Egyptian coins. They then went back to their positions and continued, when necessary, to shoot to kill each other – to me, this was somewhat reminiscent of the German and British troops in World War I coming out of the trenches into no-man's-land to drink a toast together to Christmas and the New Year, play a game of soccer, and then return to the trenches to continue the carnage.

Boredom remained the biggest problem we had in Africa. We were confined to a small area that we never left except to go out to the platoons, and when we weren't on guard there was little to occupy our time other than to sleep. I had made sure to equip myself with several novels to read, and although I had plenty of time at my disposal, I must somehow have been in some sort of a state of lethargy, because I ended by reading virtually nothing while I was in Africa. The army did what it could to alleviate the boredom, of which the most important was to send entertainers around to the different units, and this was a real treat for us. First and foremost, all the different regiments in *Tzahal* have entertainment groups. In times of emergency, they do not restrict their performing to their own regiments – they are simply sent from unit to unit to give forty-five to sixty-minute performances. I spoke to some of them and they told me that they were exhausted by their daily travelling in jeeps or command cars, as well of course by the numerous performances they had to give. In addition to the regimental entertainment groups there were famous singers or musicians, and we always particularly looked forward to their visits. (I remember one musician who played the musical saw – in fact, a terrible screeching sound, but certainly worth listening to when you have nothing else to do in Africa.) International entertainers like Danny Kaye and Isaac Stern also came to Israel to show their support and entertain the troops, but we were never lucky enough to see anyone of that stature.

Newspapers, magazines and transistor radios were sent to us, and we gained a strong sense that the folks at home really cared about us. Schools also arranged for the children to write us letters, and we would reply. Lisa, a young cousin of mine, had immigrated to Israel not long before the outbreak of the war, and she was in elementary school. All the children in her class would write letter after letter to their relatives in the army but, being new to the country, Lisa did not have anyone to write to except for her cousin David, and she and I corresponded throughout this period; I became her personal soldier. Other people in her class also wrote to me, and I found it really sweet and touching to read their letters. Another source of distraction, albeit less pure than school children's letters, were the packages of old *Playboy* magazines that would arrive from time to time and which were, of course, a big hit.

One day, by chance, I found a partial solution to my boredom problem. I was chatting with our battalion doctor and with our brigade doctor, who was on a visit to our *ta'agad*. They were asking me what I did in civilian life, and I explained to them that I taught Applied Linguistics and English as a Foreign Language at the Hebrew University. All of a sudden our doctor's face lit up:

"Have you ever done any editing?" he asked excitedly.

"Sure I have," I replied.

"Would you be willing to edit some articles that we have written?" he asked.

I was very familiar with the type of editing that they were asking for – they were both specialists in the same area of lipid research, and were both also appointed to a university medical school. Moreover, they had both spent an extended period abroad, so that their English was good, although not good enough to allow them to submit scholarly research articles to an English-speaking journal without their being edited.

Now this may look at first glance like a case of *force majeure*. After all, the battalion doctor was the officer to whom I reported, and the brigade doctor was even higher than that. But, in fact, the relationships

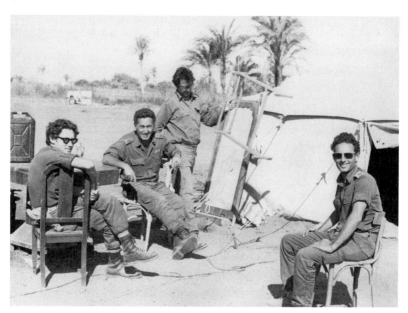

Preparing to edit the two doctors' articles in the middle of the desert. They (seated left) look happy and confident, but I (standing) look decidedly apprehensive.

were such that I certainly could have refused. However I jumped at the opportunity, seeing this as a way of activating my gray cells, idle for far too long. I edited at least two articles for these doctors during that time, and still have a photograph of this amazing scene, with the three of us sitting in the middle of nowhere, in Africa, working on one of them.

We did not have any access to what *Tzahal* deemed a healthy water supply. The premise *Tzahal* worked on was that all the water in the area was infested with bilharzia, and the order was that we were under no circumstances to have contact with any water from an Egyptian source. The area where we were stationed was very primitive, and there were no water taps, so the danger was mainly from contact with water in the Sweetwater Canal. Some of our units were located on one side of this canal, and some on the other, and there were few crossing points. As a result, some of the soldiers built a sort of a raft-cum-ferry to get across. You stood on it and hauled the raft across by pulling a rope on a pulley. But this was a rickety structure, and there was always a danger of falling into the water. An even more serious danger was of a vehicle rolling into the canal because of the soft, unmarked shoulders of the sand road along it, as it was not always easy to see where the road ended and the shoulder began. We had one instance in which a jeep belonging to my battalion moved to the side of the road because of an oncoming vehicle, and the shoulder gave way. The jeep rolled over into the canal. There were four people in the jeep, and they all miraculously escaped injury. However, they all got wet, and as a result were all airlifted to a civilian hospital immediately – which will give you some indication of how seriously *Tzahal* took the bilharzia threat.

Everyone kept as far from the local water as possible. But we also needed a water source for cooking, drinking and washing/showering. At the beginning, the only sources we had were twenty-liter containers that were trucked in from Israel, and they were in very short supply. In fact one day during our first week in Africa I was dying for a shower, and a friend and I decided that we would 'shower' each other. We stripped naked and, with a small tin, poured water over each other's heads and showered that way. Unfortunately for us, just as we were showering, one of our battalion majors walked by, and he was livid. He began to shout and scream at us about wasting precious water and, of course, he was absolutely correct, as there had been an explicit ban on doing what we did. While we were not actually punished, we were made painfully aware that we should not be doing what we were doing, and indeed felt suitably guilty and stupid when we were caught.

Not long after we arrived the army erected two large water towers, each of which held a good reserve of water, and these were filled by water trucked in by tankers from Israel. We were officially told that we were allowed to shower. But ... it was all very well and good to *allow* us to shower, but there were no showers. So a few of the more handy soldiers decided that they were going to build one. They began by scrounging and improvising parts, and within about four days we had a shower that worked in the following way. There was a container set up about eight feet from the ground, and out of it came a piece of hose, with a tap-device to close off the flow. You may have noted that there was no mention of the container being attached to any water source. What is more, it was getting colder by the day while we were in Africa, so that we not only needed a water source, but a hot water source. So when you wanted to shower, what you had to do was first to borrow the paraffin cooker and a very large cooking pot which, thankfully, armies have in abundance, and then heat a pot of water. The paraffin cooker was like one of those one-fire, very weak heat camping stoves, and heating a large pot of water took well over an hour. Since this was not enough water for a decent shower, we heated the water to almost boiling and then mixed it with cold water to get a reasonable amount of warm water. Once the water was hot, you took it and a container of cold water, stood on a structure that our ingenious friends had built, and poured some of each into the elevated container. Then you stripped and began showering. When the container became empty, you repeated the process. This whole showering ritual took at least two hours from start to finish, but let me tell you that it was worth every minute of it. Not only did you have a hot shower, which is something heavenly especially when living as we were, but it also filled the best part of half a day. Unfortunately, on the same day that the second floor of our building was destroyed, one of the two water towers was blown to pieces, and water rationing began all over again.

If so far I have made little reference to the food we were given in Africa, maybe that is because in some ways I have tried to block it out of my mind. One of the major disadvantages of having moved up from being a platoon to a battalion medic in the *ta'agad* was the fact that the *ta'agad* is part of Headquarters Company. This means that the small *ta'agad* group of seven or eight medics, the doctor, radio man and ambulance driver are not 'independent.' They are part of a much larger group of soldiers – a company of about a hundred – and for many things in day-to-day army life we were subject to the sergeant major of the company and not just to the doctor. And the company sergeant major of Headquarters Company was not a very pleasant or a very wise individual, and one moreover whose baleful influence extended as far as the preparation of food, on which it had an unfortunate impact. Being in Headquarters Company we ate food prepared in bulk by army cooks, whereas on the front line the soldiers were divided into units that lived and guarded together in groups that seldom exceeded twenty, and they cooked their own food. Consequently they were able to be really creative, and with the ample time we all had on our hands, they prepared some remarkably tasty meals consisting of such things as deep fried *luf* patties.

What was *luf*? Armies are famous, or should I say infamous, for their food, although I must say that *Tzahal* has always done its utmost to provide reasonable food, even in the battle rations that we were given. In Africa, though, there was a major problem: we had no refrigeration, and so virtually all food was canned. Now it so happened that for several years *Tzahal* had been using a fatty, canned meat loaf. On the label, the word 'loaf' was transliterated into Hebrew and should have been rendered as 'lof' (pronounced 'lawf'). However, because modern Hebrew does not print the vowel diacritics, it came to be read as *luf* – rhyming with 'woof.' But the real problem was not the mispronunciation of the word, but the taste of the meat – it was awful! I can only assume that it was equivalent to the spam that was so infamous in Second World War stories of the British army. The only difference was that *luf* was kosher, of course, but that did not help to improve its taste. If you have conjured up notions of bully beef let me hasten to disillusion you – *luf* was *far* worse! Bully beef was an attempt at providing stewed meat. *Luf*, on the other hand, was processed ground meat. And in Headquarters Company, in which army cooks cooked for over a hundred people, the *luf* that we were served was simply unpalatable. Perhaps I am being unfair – it was palatable for about a week, but after that we just stopped going to lunch, the main meal, because we knew what awaited us. There were one or two occasions on which *Tzahal* flew in some fresh produce, and such occasions were like feasts. The highlight was little plastic bags of chocolate-flavored milk, known in Israel as 'shoko.' Refrigeration of this delicious chocolate milk was never a problem, since it never lasted long enough to require storage.

It did not take long for us to find some sort of a solution to the *luf* problem. We withdrew to our *ta'agad* group, and began bringing food from home. But this, too, was limited by the refrigeration problem. We quickly 'trained' our wives in what to buy for us to take back, and this included such things as instant soups that only required that you add water, cheese in tubes, and the like. And then I had a brainwave.

From my first leave I brought back what in South Africa we had called a 'jaffle iron.' This was a primitive, non-electric toasted sandwich maker. It had two long handles like those you find on barbecue tongs, and at the end of each was a circular, saucer-like piece of metal. These were hinged together, making a closed space into which to insert the pieces of bread. Then all you had to do was to hold this over any heat source, and in due course you had a toasted sandwich, as tasty as any sandwiches made by electric sandwich makers today. The only snag was – what should we put onto the bread? After all, at home, one would put such things as cheese, or cheese and tomato, or egg, none of which was available to us. We became very inventive, and in no time were making such things as sardine jaffles, *luf* jaffles (delicious, actually), jam jaffles, mackerel jaffles, and more. All of these fillings were available in abundance in tins. The jaffles were an instant success! We made them using the same little stove that we used to heat water for showering, and we each averaged two jaffles per meal. Before long news of our jaffles spread, and soon we found ourselves cooking for more than just the *ta'agad*. But no one minded as there was always plenty of both food and time, so our jaffle banquets became major social events.

Getting clean clothes was also a major preoccupation, and while in Africa I had a scary incident relating to changing my clothes. Reservists in *Tzahal* are not issued with permanent uniforms for which they are responsible; instead, on being called up, we were given a set of what was known as 'work uniform' (as opposed to 'dress uniform'). These were army uniforms of national servicemen who had completed their service and who, on being discharged, had handed back their uniforms to the quartermaster. As a result, they were pretty well worn by the time we got them, and it was always touch and go as to whether you would find anything that fitted you, particularly if you were on the larger side in terms of height or girth. We were each issued with one pair of pants and one shirt, which we wore day and night for a full week, after which a clean consignment arrived and we could go and exchange our dirty, or should I say filthy, clothes for clean ones.

All medics were issued with six phials of morphine. We were required to keep these in our shirt pockets at all times, and it was made very clear to us from the day we were taught about morphine in the medic's course that if we lost one of these phials, or could not account for one, we would be put on military trial immediately. Well, one slow day in Africa, we were called to go and change our clothes – always a delight, I must say. When my turn came, I was given a clean set, and took great delight in parting with the smelly, sweaty set of the previous week. I threw them on the pile, along with hundreds of others. About an hour later, I suddenly realized that I had not removed the morphine from my pocket. I rushed to the room where the laundry had been issued, offering up a prayer as I ran along that the dirty clothes had not yet been taken away. Luckily for me they were still there, and I was allowed to sift through all the hundreds of smelly shirts till I found my morphine. An unpleasant task but, in view of the fate that awaited me if my search proved unsuccessful, well worth it, believe me.

As was the case in other stints of army service, although we were so different and came from so many and such different backgrounds, our *ta'agad* group became a 'band' – a group of friends, and we got to know each other well, getting along splendidly considering our different backgrounds and interests. One matter, however, was to drive something of a wedge between the *chovshim* in the *ta'agad*. One day, without any warning or preparation, we were informed that the army had awarded some promotions. Among them was the promotion of two of the corporals, one being me, to the rank of sergeant. As I explained, rank made absolutely no difference and we wore no marking to show it, nor were our duties, living conditions or anything else determined by whether we were sergeants or corporals. We were all equals as *chovshim* of the *ta'agad*, and I don't even think it made any difference to our army pay; if it did, then the difference was infinitesimal. However, when this news of promotions was announced, it unleashed all sorts of horrible jealousies, and the two of us became the objects of resentment for our promotions over which we had no control whatsoever, while those who had been overlooked for promotion felt left out and held us responsible. It reminded me of John Steinbeck's famous 1947 story, *The Pearl*, in which a Mexican Indian pearl diver finds a pearl on the beach. Far from improving his life, it causes such fights and jealousies among his family that he ends up throwing it back into the sea. I would gladly have done the same with my sergeant's stripes.

But I also made new friends in Africa, and one person I met for the first time was a Jerusalemite named David. When I saw him I guessed who he was, because David is the spitting image of his older brother, Michael, who had taught high school with me a few years earlier. David was also a medic, but he was in a field hospital to which we evacuated our wounded. One day he arrived at our battalion aid station to carry out some task or other, we began chatting, and I learned that he was a doctoral student at Oxford, and that he had returned to Israel to serve in the war. I told him that I was being considered for a scholarship to do my Ph.D. in the coming academic year, and that more than likely I would choose Edinburgh University if I got it. We made a pact: if he and I survived the war, and I got the scholarship, we would meet the following Passover either at his home in Oxford or in Edinburgh for the Passover Seder. Well, we both survived, David returned to Oxford, I was awarded the scholarship, and in the summer of 1974 Jenny and I, with our two daughters, went off to Scotland so that I could pursue graduate studies in linguistics. The following Spring, as Passover approached, I made contact with David, and he, and his wife and baby son came to stay with us in Edinburgh, and there, true to our pact, we celebrated Passover together. It was a thrilling moment, linking Jerusalem, Ismailia and Edinburgh and the friendship that had grown between us. We had hit it off from the moment we met, largely because he, like me, was clearly a reluctant soldier, but nevertheless still doing his duty with dedication.

Tzahal has always been a compassionate army, and no, I do not think that is an oxymoron. This compassion certainly extends to the recognition that it is a peoples' army made up largely of reservists who, like me, would have greatly preferred to have been at home. Consequently, leave was a very precious commodity, and every effort was made to send as many of us home on leave as often as possible. However actually getting to Jerusalem was no simple matter, as we were very far away. Officers were automatically entitled to flights to Tel Aviv in Hercules military aircraft from the commandeered Egyptian military airfield at Fa'id, while those of us who were not officers were provided with buses that ran daily from Africa to Tel Aviv. The only catch was that it took about 12 hours to get from where we were by bus to Tel Aviv, and then you had to hitchhike to Jerusalem. We were allowed to go to the airfield and see whether there was any space in the planes, and after all the officers were on board every effort was made to fit as many of us in as possible. The flight itself, if you were lucky enough to be on it, was a highly uncomfortable experience, as these transport planes did not have seats, so we sat on our packs on the floor, with our legs crossed so as to take up as little room as possible. I managed to get a flight twice, and it was really comical. Once the officers were seated we were told we could board, upon which we all made a mad dash for the plane lest we be left behind and compelled to travel by bus, and in no time the plane was full. Or so we thought. It reminded me of sitting on the floor in the school hall for Assembly. At that moment, the pilot came into the passenger area and shouted: "There are still a lot of soldiers waiting to board. Move right up!" We all squashed together, and probably another 30-40 soldiers squeezed onto the plane. The flight took about an hour, as I recall, and no one minded the discomfort – it sure as hell beat 12 hours in a bus through the desert.

Going home was magical! We were usually given about five days' leave, which meant at least three days at home, and we cherished every moment of it. Yet, when I returned home, it was a bittersweet moment: my younger daughter, Noa, who was not yet three, did not recognize me. Of course it didn't take her long to warm to me, but that was a nasty and unsettling experience, yet another grim reminder of the costs of war.

When we came on leave, it quickly became apparent that we were importing the Egyptian fleas to Jerusalem, and word spread rapidly that, although we were unaware of it, our clothes were infested with them. By the time my turn for my first leave arrived I knew of this problem, so on arrival at our apartment, instead of rushing in and flinging my arms around Jenny and the girls as I wanted to, I stood on the back porch where the laundry was done and shed my clothes, which went straight into the washing machine.

Over the time that we were together in the *ta'agad*, despite the jealousy and ill feeling over the promotions, our small group became and remained close. For example, since communication between Africa and Jerusalem was extremely limited, days would often go by without our being able to make contact with our loved ones. As a result, we developed a system whereby whenever one of us went on leave, he would call the wives of the whole group and send love, and would of course bring back anything that any of the wives wanted to send. This always included creative fillings for the jaffles.

Israel is a family-conscious society, as indeed Jews have always been wherever they have lived throughout the centuries and around the world. I am not sure how such a trait develops; perhaps partly a result of their rejection in so many places by the local non-Jewish population. In any event, this very positive feature has been transported to modern Israel intact, and Israelis place a high premium on family and close family ties – more so, I believe, than in North America – and this is reflected in all facets of society. It is paradoxical that, at least at the surface level, Israelis appear to be uncaring and rough with each other in their interpersonal relationships. However, when you scratch the surface, you find a deeply caring society, and one which closes ranks and is at its best in times of trouble. It is therefore not surprising that we spent a lot of time talking to each other about our wives and our children, sharing the things we read in letters – this child cut its first tooth, that one grazed his knee, and so on. In a very short time we came to know all about each others' families, and when we called the wives while on leave would ask things like, "Is your son over his cold?" and "How is your daughter enjoying day-care?"

Now in our group there was one man, Yehuda, who talked incessantly about his daughter. He only had the one daughter, and clearly she was the pride of his life, the very apple of his eye. He used to drone on and on about her. I remember so clearly him receiving a letter and then, bursting with pride and excitement, telling a few of us that his daughter was starting to learn ballet – she was about six. Shortly after that, I went on leave, and duly called all the wives. When I reached Yehuda's wife I asked her, "How is your daughter enjoying her dancing lessons?" There was a long pause and then she replied, "We don't have a daughter. We don't have any children."

While on leave, I went to visit numerous people who had been wounded in the war and were recovering in a military rehabilitation hospital near Tel Aviv. All but one of those that I visited were ex-students of mine from the Hebrew University High School. As I had left the school in the summer of 1969, and it was now early 1974, this meant that these kids had been through their army service, with many of them signing on for extra service and becoming officers, serving in the thick of several battles in this war. It was tragic seeing these young people in their early twenties. Two of the boys had suffered burst ear drums from explosions, and were having a great deal of difficulty hearing what was being said. They thought it highly amusing that they had to shout at each other, but my heart broke. One of the wounded was a young girl I had taught who had been caught in a relatively forward position in Sinai when the war began, and had been badly injured in both legs, and only miraculous work by a team of orthopedic surgeons was able to save her legs. But her walking was permanently affected, and her legs remained appallingly scarred. This beautiful young woman told me she would never wear a skirt again.

One of the people I visited in that same hospital was Meir, the American from our unit, who had lost an arm and part of his face and nose in the Katyusha attack. When I visited him I found him in a private room, which puzzled me as he was no more severely wounded than many of the soldiers I'd seen in the large communal wards. And then he explained that, being a native speaker of English, the army used him for some public relations work when Americans on solidarity visits were brought to the hospital. He thought this was hilarious.

"Open the closet," he told me.

As I did, hundreds of packets of cigarettes cascaded onto the floor. And Meir did not even smoke. They had been given to him by the solidarity visitors, who arrived in a steady stream to visit him.

At the time of the war, Meir was a doctoral student in the social sciences. His injuries were visible to all – both his seriously disfigured face, and the sleeve of his pajamas covering the short stump of what had been an arm, flapping uselessly when he spoke. He definitely had a wicked, black sense of humor, and the first thing he asked me was, "Did you give my arm an appropriate burial?" He told me with great pride that his favorite trick, when people asked him what he did before the war, was to answer, "I was a concert pianist." This was, of course, total nonsense, but he loved to watch the reaction of the visitors when he said it. He laughed and laughed as he told me this story.

I think they call this a defense mechanism, because the end of the story about Meir is, however, even sadder than this, and bereft of all humor. He never returned to his studies, nor did he ever work again – deep inside him were injuries to his psyche which were far more damaging than the horrific external injuries. In short, his life was ruined.

A dimension of this whole reservist soldier situation that is seldom given adequate attention is how those that we left behind at home coped with the situation. I won't attempt to generalize, but will merely describe what it was like for Jenny, whose unflagging love and support throughout this time gave me all the strength I needed.

You might wonder, for instance, how we managed financially. I have several times commented on the uniqueness of *Tzahal* and, indeed, of Israel, and the way in which this problem is handled is, in my opinion, most impressive. As a salaried employee at the university, a monthly sum was always deducted as an obligatory payment to the National Insurance Institute. Whenever I was called up to serve in *miluim*, the university would continue to pay my salary *in full* with no delays or deductions, and would claim this back from National Insurance, so we did not suffer financially at all. But there remained the question of what happened with our work. In my case, teaching in the English Department at The Hebrew University and moonlighting doing similar work one day a week in Beersheba at the fledgling Ben Gurion University of the Negev, my work inevitably did suffer.

Although the academic year in Israel normally opens ten days to two weeks after Yom Kippur, in 1973 the university authorities sensibly decided to postpone the opening of the year by a couple of months because so many students and faculty were in the army. The year finally opened, without me of course, around December, and I only returned to work in the middle of March, at which point I did the best I could to cover as much as possible of my courses in the time remaining. However, committed though I am to my work and to my profession, the importance of this paled into oblivion in comparison with everything that was going on around us.

Unfortunately, as I learned from my friends, the situation for self-employed people was far more problematic, and I would hear them complain constantly about this when we were in the army. In addition to the actual compensation they received from National Insurance, which they claimed was below what it should be, there was the problem of losing customers. Several of the people I served with were in very small businesses or workshops. For example, two men had just opened a garage together, another had a small truck and made his living bringing produce from the wholesale market to the vendors in the Machane Yehuda market, and one was a carpenter who worked with one employee making such items as built-in closets and bedroom sets. The problem that they faced was that their customers generally would not or could not wait for them, and took their business elsewhere. In short, they simply lost their clientele, most of whom never returned, and I know of several men who became bankrupt as a result of the war.

True, Jenny and I did not suffer financially, but Jenny had to bear other burdens, and these were significant. At that time she was working at the Jewish National and University Library. This was hard enough with the two little girls but, as fate would have it, precisely in the 1973-74 academic year she took a graduate library science degree as well. We knew from the outset, without ever dreaming that there was going to be a war, that this would at best prove to be a crowded and difficult year for us, and that I would have to play a more significant role in the housekeeping and child-care. Little did we know that Anwar Sadat of Egypt had other plans for me. But when the war broke out we decided that Jenny must still carry on with her plan, because without it she would be unable to advance her career. What is more, we knew that there was a chance that the following year we would be going overseas for me to do my Ph.D., and that the librarian's qualification would be crucial for Jenny in finding a good job.

And then, to crown everything, my father became very ill. In December he had to have prostate surgery, which was bad enough. But around the same time, the doctors also diagnosed that he was suffering from a type of degenerative brain disease. This led to a serious loss of small motor skills, making it difficult for him to perform certain even quite basic functions. This meant that my mother had to carry this burden, and she could not carry it alone. Jenny now stepped in and helped them in every way imaginable – all this in spite of the myriad of other things she had to do – with whatever needed to be done in their apartment. But more importantly, Jenny now stood rock solid beside my parents providing them – or more correctly, my mother – with the kind of emotional and moral support that they had lavished on us all these years. We were extremely close with all our parents, and Jenny helped my parents with the love of a deeply devoted daughter. Her mother all this time was living in the Tel Aviv area and working full time, which restricted the amount that she was able to do to help except on weekends, leaving Jenny to cope almost alone.

In January the doctors decided that my father had to have an invasive test to determine what exactly the problem was. They warned us that this test was dangerous and could even be life threatening. And there I was, making jaffles in Africa. I was frantic. I not only desperately wanted to be there with my family, but I also needed to be there to share the responsibility with Jenny. I turned, once again, to Dudu. Dudu, the man who had been my company commander in the Six Day War, and whom I so admired. By this stage Dudu had been promoted to battalion second-in-command – luckily for me, as I was now attached to Headquarters Company, which brought me into close and daily contact with him. I asked to see him, explained my situation, and asked for special leave to go to Jerusalem. Once more, he proved to be the ultimate "mensch" (fine, decent human being).

"So may I go?" I asked.

"Of course you can go," he said, "When is the procedure being done?"

"On Wednesday," I replied.

"Then you can go on Tuesday."

"But when do I have to be back?" I asked.

Dudu took a piece of paper out of his pocket and wrote something down on it and handed it to me: "Here is my home phone number. I will be home on leave on Friday afternoon. Call me at home and report to me how your father is doing, and I will decide then when you must go back."

My eyes filled with tears. I have never before or since encountered such compassion and understanding from a person in a military position of authority.

My father had the test on the Wednesday, and came through it without suffering any ill effects. On the Friday afternoon, I called Dudu at home and reported to him that my father had come through the test safely.

"So do you think you can return to duties on Sunday?" he asked.

"Definitely," I replied. And that is what I did.

Against all these odds, Jenny completed her library degree that year, the first step on what has since been a fine career in librarianship. Whoever coined the term "the weaker sex" for women was sorely mistaken. Jenny's strength of character and cool composure throughout this traumatic period is living proof of the sheer folly of applying that term. This was a terribly difficult time for her, and she came through with flying colors. I never heard her complain about anything – she was always serene, calm, and lovingly in control.

At the same time it was, obviously, also a nightmare period for my mother. I say for my mother and not for my parents, because my father's illness made him somewhat unaware of day-to-day needs and pressures. During the time I was in Africa he also stopped working, and took early medical retirement. This posed no problem for him, but put even more pressure on my mother, because now he was at home all day and had to be cared for, while she still had a full time job.

The situation militarily remained virtually static throughout that long, drawn-out time I was in Africa. I call it static but, as I have already said, that does not mean that it was particularly safe. By static I mean that there were no troop advances or withdrawals by either side. And the Egyptian Third Army remained encircled and besieged by *Tzahal*.

Politically, however, there was a great deal of activity, particularly at the international level. Richard Nixon was the U.S. President at the time, and Henry Kissinger the Secretary of State, and they were both doing their best for Israel, both publicly and certainly behind the scenes. Having political views that lean to the left of center, I was always in favor of a Democrat President in the U.S. However Nixon, the Republican, proved to be very good for Israel. There was clear cut evidence of staunch support from Nixon and the United States – witness some remarkable photographs of gigantic military cargo planes coming in to land at Lod International Airport. On one occasion, I actually saw one of these planes when I went to the airport to try and get a flight back to Africa after leave.

Henry Kissinger embarked on his shuttle diplomacy, traveling between Damascus, Cairo and Jerusalem, sometimes backwards and forwards the very same day, trying to help the sides find viable ways to disentangle themselves without losing face, without endangering their soldiers, and without this constituting a step that might be interpreted as weakness at home or by the other side.

Kissinger shuttled, and we waited. And we waited. And we waited. All we wanted at this stage, in the early months of 1974, was to know that there was some sort of agreement which would enable us to go home. In fact, all we wanted was a *date* – a date when we would be leaving Africa, so that we could begin counting down the remaining days.

To be serving and not to know when this would come to an end was stressful indeed for us and, of course, for our loved ones at home. You will recall that I said that whenever we were in *miluim* we used to count the days left to serve; now, being in a war situation, we were unable to do this, and although this might sound unimportant, it was not so to us.

Finally, in early February, a troop disengagement agreement was reached between Israel and Egypt: both sides would pull back from the areas they had captured during the fighting – Israel from Africa, and Egypt from the piece of land on the eastern side of the Suez Canal where the Third Army was trapped – with a schedule of dates by which the withdrawals would be completed by both sides. Finally, we were going home! Even if we didn't know the precise date, this was more than sufficient cause for great excitement as we waited anxiously to learn when exactly we would be leaving Africa. However, as luck would have it, *Tzahal* decided for its own reasons that the withdrawal would begin in the town of Suez at the southern end of the captured enclave, ending with the withdrawal of our unit from the area closest to Ismailia in the north. Although envious of those serving nearer Suez because they would be home ahead of us, and disappointed that we would be the last to withdraw, at least now we had a date to count backwards from, and that made us very happy. In addition, the security situation locally calmed right down once the plans were in place, and the nightly shooting came to an almost complete halt.

We began to ponder: How do we celebrate the countdown – the thing we had been watching and waiting for? We decided to make a chart, and each morning to scratch off the day that had just passed. I had a brainwave. I made my suggestion to the rest of the medics and they jumped at it. We painted a huge calendar on the wall of the room we slept in. We did not have any paint, so we used what is called in Israel 'brilliant green,' something we had in abundance. 'Brilliant green' is iodine used in the cleaning of wounds, and it is indeed a wonderfully bright, emerald green color. (In some countries bright red mercurochrome, or bright purple gentian violet – also iodine based – are variants of brilliant green.) We had no paintbrushes, so we used 'Q-tips,' of which we also had copious quantities in the *ta'agad*. We painted a huge calendar on the largest wall of our room with each square, representing a day, being about four inches square. At that point there were about thirty days to go. In the top left-hand square we wrote 'Africa' and an arrow pointing rightwards, and in the bottom right-hand square we wrote 'Jerusalem.' And in each square we wrote the date in small letters, and the number of days left in large. But how to check off the days? This was my moment of genius. We decided that each morning we would assemble at the chart, and would take it in turns deleting the day that had just passed by

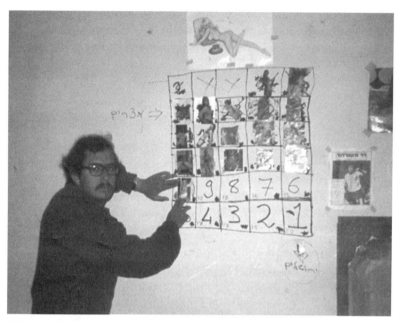

The demob pin-up calendar. Early 1974.

covering the square with the pin-up chosen by the medic whose turn it was. Both *Tzahal* and Israel at this time received munificent support from the United States, and one of the forms that this took was large packages of old copies of *Playboy*. The rumor was that these packages were personally arranged by Pat Nixon, the First Lady, and we were happy to accept this as fact. However, to be honest, we never actually found out who sent them. Living as we did in the pre-political correctness age, we were delighted to receive them, whoever the sender might be. As we did not have glue to stick the pin-ups to the wall we used Vaseline, of which again there was no shortage.

The fame of our chart soon spread, and as the days went by more and more soldiers from other units based with us used to join us for the pin-up ceremony. We loved it, but unfortunately like all famous frescoes it was not portable so we had to leave it as a legacy for the Egyptians. All I have to show for it is a color slide of the chart that I took when it was about half way through.

Once the disengagement agreement was in place, night firing and sniping stopped, and it became much safer near the line. So some of us had a great idea: we went to one of the senior officers and suggested to him that we bring our wives down to Africa to visit us for one night. What we suggested was that we would all chip in and charter a full size bus, with the wives leaving Jerusalem very early one morning so that they would arrive in Africa in the late afternoon. They would stay until early the following afternoon, when the bus would set out to take them back to Jerusalem. Somewhat to our surprise permission was granted, and we moved into action. In no time we had enough people signed up to fill the bus, and we began planning the logistics. We set a date, and began notifying our wives and arranging accommodation. We were told that the wives would not be allowed to sleep on the line where our platoons were based, but would sleep at Headquarters Company, where the *ta'agad* was stationed. There was a large room in the stone building, normally used as a dining room, and the wives were told to bring sleeping bags and sleep there. We also had to arrange a pass for the bus. The entire western sector of the Sinai Peninsula was a military zone and not open to civilians, so special permission was needed for the bus and all the wives to pass beyond the checkpoint.

On the home front, there were also logistics to be worked out. In order to come, Jenny, like so many of the other wives, had to arrange time off work and plan for our little girls. My mother, despite having a full time job herself, stepped right in as usual, and looked after the girls so that Jenny could participate. Somehow, when it came to this kind of request, the answer was always an unhesitating "yes," and somehow she worked it out with her employers.

The night before the wives were due to arrive, I managed to arrange that I would be the medic who would go in a command car to meet the bus at the checkpoint and accompany it all the way to where we were stationed. Excitement was at fever pitch as we – a driver, an officer and I, the token medic – set off to meet the wives. It was quite a long distance back to the checkpoint and we were not at all sure exactly how long the bus would take to get there. We had to drive south in Africa to where the crossing-point was and then a long way east across the Sinai Peninsula, so we set out in very good time. In fact we set out much too early – we were simply too eager – and we ended up spending about three hours in the middle of the desert waiting for the bus. While we

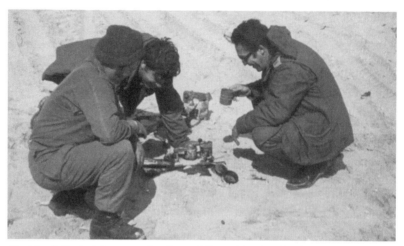

Cooking luf *to while away the time while waiting in the desert for our wives' arrival.*

waited, we made a little fire and heated up tinned *luf* and ate it with some bread. But this time we did not mind the *luf* at all. Finally, the bus arrived, and the thrill of greeting everyone, and specially of seeing Jenny, was enormous.

We drove down to the Suez Canal and, while still on the eastern side before crossing, took the wives to see an Israeli *mutzav*, which had been overrun by the Egyptians in the first days of the war, and subsequently abandoned. It was a very moving experience to realize that at this very spot so many of our comrades had died. Then came the actual crossing of the Canal – a very different undertaking from my original crossing during the war, when it had been on the rickety pontoon bridges of the Engineering Corps. Since then several months had passed, and *Tzahal* had trucked in hundreds and hundreds of truckloads of earth and stone and dumped them into the canal, thereby creating a solid land bridge. This land bridge, built to move troops across the canal with ease, was paved and wide enough for four tanks to travel alongside each other. The reason for this was that there was constant danger throughout this period that our force on the western side of the Canal could be cut off from the rest of the army and from its supply lines – just as we had done to the Egyptian Third Army on the eastern side of the Canal – and this bridge had been built to prevent such a thing happening. We got out of the bus at the bridge and walked across, an exciting moment recorded in two photos I have of Jenny and me standing on the bridge road half way across the Canal. We had a real sense that we were taking part in a historic event. And Jenny is clearly one of the few women who crossed that land bridge and visited Africa under Israeli occupation.

From there, we went to an abandoned Egyptian *mutzav* opposite the Israeli one we had just visited, and saw how clearly the Egyptians could see everything on the Israeli side, and just how vulnerable our soldiers had been. And then we drove to the village where we were stationed. Jenny and the wives were fascinated by the villages that we passed through, but disturbed by the poverty and the fact that the houses, or hovels, were made of mud. Jenny was particularly fascinated by the dovecots, also made of mud, which existed in each village. The doves, we learned, were an important source of protein, particularly as there was no electricity in these villages so that refrigeration was a problem, making it hard to keep fresh food.

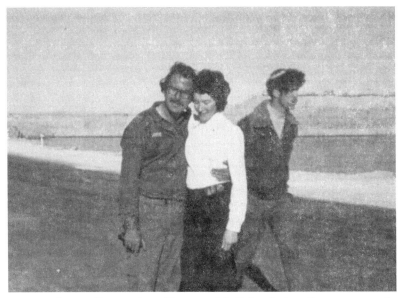

Jenny and I standing on the military road built by the Israeli army across the Suez Canal. With the eventual reopening of the Suez Canal, the road was demolished.

On arrival at Headquarters Company, all the husbands from the different platoons whose wives were on the trip were waiting, and the scene of the reunion was one that remains with me still. True, we had all had leave, but to be able actually to show our wives where we had been serving, and how we had been living, was in many ways deeply moving. It was also strangely revealing to see and get to know many of the wives. After all, we were a mixed group, thrown together by circumstance to live and work for a common endeavor. Moreover, wearing uniform is an excellent leveler, and meeting the wives in their normal civilian clothing somehow heightened how different and disparate we really were.

Meeting the other medics' wives was a particularly strange experience. We had all heard so much about each of them, but had not met most of them. The differences in our backgrounds had long since ceased to matter. But all of a sudden, confronted with the wives, these differences all came to the fore, not only evidenced by the type of clothing they wore, but also by the type of food they brought for us. Yet in spite of these differences, we made an agreement there and then that the *ta'agad* team would hold a party in Jerusalem soon after we were demobilized.

Soon after the wives' arrival it began getting dark, so we got organized for supper. We had planned a festive dinner – army style – and social evening. All the men whose wives were on the bus were allowed to stay at Headquarters Company and attend the festive dinner. The cooks really went out of their way to try and make this a very nice meal, and we thought that it was, although I've often wondered how the wives found it. I know that Jenny was thrilled and perfectly happy with the effort that had been made, although it wasn't a gourmet feast by even the most generous standards, despite our being so happy and proud of our efforts. People had even gone out and found a few shrubs and put them in empty bottles to decorate the tables. To be precise there were no tables, so what we used as tables were things like old doors or planks of wood, propping them up on boxes.

Jenny is very easy-going and uncomplaining, and she was just delighted with everything, even the meal we served them based on the same canned foods, including the dreaded *luf* we had been eating for so many months. However, this was not true of all the wives. One of the things that astounded me was that there were quite a few women who did not stop complaining from the time we met the bus until the time we said goodbye to them. They complained about the long and bumpy bus ride; they complained about the meal; and they complained vociferously about the sleeping conditions. I really wonder how their poor husbands felt. After all, this was the best that we were able to offer them, and to be a little uncomfortable for one night and to eat the food we ate for one meal was a small price to pay in order to be able to share in our unique experience.

After supper – I hesitate to call it dinner – we cleared away the tables and made room for everyone to sit and take part in a sing-song. Our battalion commander, a regular army man, was present, and he made a brief speech welcoming the wives, telling them a little about what we had been doing and going through. After that we settled down to an evening of community singing and humor, and it was truly a lot of fun. The husbands then had to return to their positions, and the chairs were cleared away and mattresses put on the floor for the wives. Once again, there was much loud complaint from certain wives, which reached a shrill crescendo the following morning when several of them informed us that they had been bitten by fleas during the night! Well, *Tzahal* really went out of its way to make this stay memorable, and none of us was too sympathetic. Frankly, I think certain of the women should never have come. After all, it was not obligatory.

Breakfast was served on the line at one of our platoons, and once again tremendous efforts had been made to welcome the wives in style. I mentioned earlier that the area we were in had orange groves. Well, by this time the oranges had ripened, and a group of soldiers had gone and picked hundreds of them, which they then squeezed *by hand* – no easy task – as we had no juicers of any kind. There must have been about 10-20 liters of freshly squeezed orange juice. It had taken them hours and hours, and the wives were very touched. The scene at breakfast was funny: there was clearly no room for the husbands to sit at the improvised tables at this outpost along with their wives, so we stood or, like overly solicitous waiters, hovered behind where our wives were sitting, and ate our food standing up. We did not mind at all.

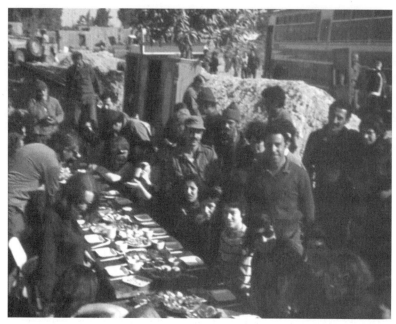

Breakfast near Ismailia for our visiting wives. Jenny is in a striped top, sitting at our improvised table.

The remainder of the morning was spent taking the wives to visit the different platoons, to see where the soldiers slept, and where they guarded. It was quiet enough by this stage, so we were allowed to take our wives right up to the front line. And then, almost as if it had been planned, as we were standing at the line in one of the outposts, along came the same group of U.N. peacekeepers again, providing a superb photo opportunity.

Finally, it was time for the wives to begin to head back to Jerusalem. After all, they had a good 12 hours of travel ahead of them on bumpy roads. Jenny and I said a rather tearful goodbye, and the bus left. This unique 20 hour interlude is something that Jenny and I cherish and talk about to this day – it gave her a real sense of where we were and what our lives had been like. I should add that Jenny thought that the chart, with the pin-ups for counting the remaining days, was hilarious.

When the wives came to visit us the end of our days in Africa was finally in sight, and we had little more than a week to wait before we withdrew. But, as is so often the way, another little disappointment awaited the *chovshim* of the *ta'agad*. We were informed that when everyone else was discharged on arrival in Jerusalem, we would still be required to stay in the army for an additional week to catalog and organize the huge amount of equipment and medical supplies in the *ta'agad* – this even included counting every aspirin, syringe, needle and bandage, and putting them all into their exact places. While this may sound somewhat petty and unnecessary, all *ta'agads* throughout *Tzahal* are arranged in precisely the same way, with precisely the same equipment, so that any *chovesh* or team of *chovshim* can take the *ta'agad* out of storage at any time, and know with certainty what they will find and not find in it, and where.

Finally, on March 8, over five months after joining my unit, our rag-tag convoy of vehicles set out from Africa for Asia. Thank God, it was over and I was able to come home safely. We were all in boisterous spirits, not even minding that much that we would have to serve an additional week, because we were allowed to do our work during the day and then to go home for the night.

As I write this and I think of that homecoming, I feel overwhelmed and tears fill my eyes. It is a feeling of great sadness for the thousands of families who were not able to enjoy the thrill of the homecoming of their loved ones – whose soldier would never return or was irreparably maimed during this terrible time in Israel's history.

We did nothing special in the family to mark my return – not a party, nor a special dinner, nor did we go away for a couple of days. I just slipped back into civilian routine, and was happy to do precisely that. Sadly, the situation with my father had deteriorated, and maybe that was why we did not mark my homecoming – I don't know. But what I do know is that my father was not coping well, and that the burden on my mother was increasing by the day. My mother was turning sixty in a few months, and was required to retire from her job in the civil service. Because of my father having taken early retirement on medical grounds, one of the first tasks that awaited me was to go to the

National Insurance Institute and arrange my mother's pension and my father's because, although he had stopped working, the paperwork still had to be sorted out.

The Israel of 1974 was much advanced over the Israel I had first encountered on my arrival in 1961, but to have to arrange these two pension matters was still nothing short of a bureaucratic nightmare. It was a job only I could do, since my father was not well enough to do it, and my mother was still working full time and looking after my father. She was, in any case, not up to handling the red tape since it was all in Hebrew, in which she was still not very proficient.

I went to the building of the National Insurance Institute early one morning, and was told that the office I needed for my father was on the first floor, while that needed for my mother was on the third floor. And I was required to take a number for each. Taking a number was a dramatic improvement in the way waiting in line functioned. In the past, you physically had to stand or sit in the order in which you were waiting, and this was not always physically possible, leading to all sorts of cheating and pushing in. Moreover, in my case, it would have been totally impossible, as I was waiting my turn for two different offices on two different floors. For my mother's pension I was number 92, and for my father's number 173. This meant a long wait, with me periodically rushing up and down between the two floors to check on how the line was progressing on each floor. God forbid that I should miss my turn for either – and people in lines of this length in places like this are not very understanding. Well, after I had been sitting for about two and a half hours, all of a sudden an office door opened and out stepped Ya'akov, one of the soldiers from Headquarters Company with whom I'd been friendly in Africa. We embraced like long lost brothers.

"What are *you* doing here?" he asked.

"I've come to arrange my mother's pension and my father's early pension," I sighed.

"Come with me," he said.

Totally ignoring the line and the looks of the people waiting, he took me into his office.

"Ettie," he shouted imperiously from his desk, "bring me the file of

Mendelsohn Hilary, and do me a favor and go down to the first floor and bring me Mendelsohn Maurice's file."

I could not believe my good luck! When Ettie returned with the two files, she was asked to make coffee for the two of us. Ya'akov went through the papers and filled out all the necessary forms. Knowing how things functioned in Israel, I had armed myself with every conceivable document that they might require. But still there was one I had omitted to bring – a letter from my father's employer verifying the start and end date of his employment. My heart sank. I knew full well what that meant – another nightmare visit. Ya'akov said to me: "Do you know the start and end dates?"

"Sure I do," I said.

"Well, give them to me and I'll sign off on the authenticity of this information. Never mind about the documentation. I trust you."

Within twenty minutes, and in spite of having failed to bring that one letter, I was out of there, with all the paperwork complete, and another hug from Ya'akov. That is what is called in Israel *protektsia* – having pull. I know that what I did was not fair to the rest of the people in the line – I jumped the line and this kind of thing infuriated me whenever it occurred but, at that moment, I was so relieved to see Ya'akov and to be treated the way he treated me, that I swallowed my principles. I rationalized it to myself by saying that everyone is doing this all the time, and not doing it would simply mean that you are a sucker. For one brief nanosecond the thought flickered through my head that all that *miluim* had been worth it.

I mentioned that we did not mark my homecoming in any special way. But that is not strictly correct – we, the members of the *ta'agad*, kept our agreement and held a party very soon after we demobilized. The party took place at the home of Yehuda, the man with the fictitious, ballet lesson-taking daughter, and the whole group assembled with their wives. But the party was not a great success. In civilian clothes, coming from our widely differing homes and lives, we suddenly found that we actually had remarkably little in common, apart from our military experience. *Tzahal*, the great leveler, was not there to do its magic. We all enjoyed ourselves, and exchanged stories and photographs, but that was the last time the group gathered as a whole. Anyway, shortly thereafter we went to Britain for three years, where I did graduate studies, after which I was assigned to a totally different arm of the military. In fact, the only member of the group that I have stayed in touch with is Tuviya, who remains a friend to this day.

Part V

FROM ISMAILIA TO TORONTO

As soon as I was demobilized, I returned to my teaching at the university. Because the university year had opened almost a trimester late it compensated by closing late, so that by the time I returned almost half of that time had passed. This meant that I had little more than half a normal academic year to teach. I went and asked my head of department what I was to do, and he gave a very sensible answer: "Cover what you can. After all, it's not been our top priority, has it?" I had to smile – this response was so different from the response of Mr. Bargur at the high school in 1967, when he reprimanded me for not turning in my grades on time. So I followed the head of department's advice, and taught only the most important parts of my usual curriculum, and I don't think that the students in my courses that year came out that much less educated.

While pleasant, it was also uncanny being back on campus. On the very first day that I was back, I taught a class in Phonetics, and the topic was 'the phoneme.' This is not an easy concept for students new to Phonetics to handle. As I walked out of the building, I was accosted by a young man with a portable tape recorder.

"Are you a student here?" he asked.

"No," I explained, "I teach here."

"Even better. I am from *Kol Yisrael* Radio, and I am doing a program on demobilized soldiers and what it is like for them to return to their civilian lives. May I interview you?"

Of course I agreed. In essence, he asked me one and one question only: "What does it feel like to be back teaching your Phonetics course after five months in the army?"

This is what I answered. "For the past five months I have been in the army, doing what I was ordered to do, serving as a medic in the front line, trying to help wounded soldiers, working to save lives, and trying myself to keep out of harm's way. I have just taught a class on the phoneme, and frankly my heart was simply not in it. I honestly couldn't care less whether they ever understand what a phoneme is or not."

I still have a recording of that interview, and I wonder how it would sound today. But one thing was certain: as much as I might have argued that things were back to normal, I still had a long way to go to regain my sense of proportion and equilibrium.

Yet somehow life did eventually return to normal. Shortly after my demobilization, I was informed that I had been awarded a three-year scholarship by The Hebrew University to go overseas to do my Ph.D. I was accepted at Edinburgh University in Scotland, whose Linguistics Department was considered at that time to be the finest in the world.

There remained the paramount question of my parents. My father's condition had deteriorated, and he needed assistance with more and more day-to-day things. My mother did a wonderful job attending to him, but she needed our help in running her home, handling accounts and any routine bureaucratic matters. After much agonizing and debate in the family, we all agreed that if we were to go to Edinburgh for three years, then my parents would have to return to South Africa, where Steve and Ami had offered to look after them and give them a loving home. Once this decision had been made, Jenny and I moved into action to sell their apartment and car and to ship their possessions before we ourselves left. And finally, in July, just a few months after I was demobilized, my parents left for Johannesburg and, a week or so later, we left for Edinburgh.

Very shortly after our arrival in Edinburgh, we learned that the city had an 'Israel Society.' This was a group of people, Jews and non-Jews, who were staunch supporters of Israel, and who got together to hear talks on the topic. The moment I made contact with them they asked me to give a talk, which I happily agreed to do. However I explained that I was merely a sergeant in the army, and so was ill equipped to offer profound commentary on the strategies or the geopolitical impact of the Yom Kippur War. I eventually titled my talk *Reflections of a Civilian at War*. I had taken our slides from Africa with me for precisely that purpose, and I gave my talk, explaining what it was like being a reserve soldier in *Tzahal*.

The lecture seemed to go over well, and after it was finished, tea was served. A woman came up to me and introduced herself:

"I found your talk very interesting. But if you think that this was a hard period for you and your family, imagine how much worse it was for us sitting in Edinburgh waiting anxiously every hour to hear the news."

I had to swallow very hard before responding in order not to be rude to her, but finally managed to say, "It must have been much worse for you." The sad part is that this foolish woman was serious.

We were overseas for just over three years. As a reserve soldier who had been abroad for an extended period, my name had been removed from my usual infantry unit and placed in a pool of soldiers awaiting reassignment on their return. Once back in Israel, I duly notified the army that I had returned, and shortly thereafter was called to a particular army base for one day. On arrival, I was interviewed by an officer who said, "I see that you are a combat medic. Well, as you know, there's a shortage right across the board, so what sort of unit would you like to be placed in?" I could not believe my ears. Was this the *Tzahal* of old that I knew? What unit would I *like* to be put into? Did I actually have a say in the matter? Things had really changed! I thought for a few minutes. I knew I did not want to return to the infantry – I had had enough of running up and down hills with a stretcher on my back, so I decided that I would opt for something totally different, and said, "The Engineering Corps." "Fine," said the officer. "We'll get in touch with you in due course. You can go home."

When I got home, I excitedly told Jenny of the wondrous changes wrought in *Tzahal*, and that, given a choice of unit in which to serve, I'd volunteered for the Engineering Corps. She was as satisfied with my choice as I was. But then I began to tell friends. "You need your head read!" they all cried, aghast. "Nobody goes into the Engineering Corps out of choice. The death and injury rate from bombs, mines and booby traps is terribly high!" Well, it was too late. I had made my request and the die was cast. I waited for my first call up to my new unit. And, sure enough, in a few weeks it arrived, and my new unit was ... the Tank Corps! So much for my choice. I was not thrilled with where I had been placed, but there was very little I had done to influence the outcome.

The amount of *miluim* any soldier does is determined by law, and the number of days are counted from April 1 – March 31 of the following year. This proved disastrous timing for me, as it meant that I could be called up to serve the maximum number of days between September 1977 and April 1978 for the 1977-78 *miluim* year, and then could be called up to do the same number again after April 1, 1978 for the 1978-79 *miluim* year. And being a medic, and given the permanent shortage of combat medics throughout *Tzahal*, that is precisely what happened. In that year, from the time we returned to the time we emigrated, which was a period of almost exactly twelve months, I served something in the order of 72 days. I was pleased to be out of the infantry, but I had to get to know a whole new group of comrades, which was the worst part of being put into a new unit. My *miluim* was dull and not very pleasant, but thankfully not dangerous.

I was initially called up for a major military exercise, which was my first encounter with the new group. But then I learned that this was a newly created unit and that no one knew anybody else, which made it much easier for all of us. The guys were nice enough, and the *miluim* was long but not too bad. One thing I really liked was the fact that the *chovshim* in the Tank Corps do not run up and down like in the infantry, but are transported behind the tanks in armored troop carriers. It was not that I was old by this stage – I was only 34 – but I'd had more than enough running around laden with equipment.

There were many people who, like me, became more and more uncomfortable with the occupation of the West Bank and Gaza and the building of settlements in the occupied territories. For many of my dear and idealistic friends the challenge became to find ways to make a difference, to participate in the demonstrations and activities of organizations like Peace Now (*Shalom Achshav*). Some, like Tuviya, worked tirelessly over the years to seek a peaceful and just solution for all the people of the region. But for me Israel had lost a lot of its uniqueness – many people had replaced idealism with materialism and, what is more, I felt that the occupation had severely damaged the moral fiber of the society. Professor Leibowitz's dismal prophecy had been proven correct. Military occupation brutalizes and, by definition, requires the occupier to do certain things and make certain decisions that are not always to the liking of liberal-minded citizens. Worst of all, I saw no indication that anything was about to improve, as Israel faced on-going Arab intransigence and unwillingness to make peace. Somehow my own belief and commitment had decreased to the point at which I and my family were ready to leave and try to rebuild our lives elsewhere. My perception was that the magic that was 'pioneering Israel,' to which I had made Aliyah in 1961, was gone. I had always felt that all the hardships and even the wars were worth it – but once I no longer felt that, then it was time to leave.

The decision to emigrate was an agonizing one, and had been coming to a head over a number of years. We loved the country and, in innumerable ways, were so happy there. We had considered not returning to Israel after our three years in Edinburgh, but then ultimately felt we had to go back. After all, we had left a country still reeling from the impact of a terrible war of survival, and I felt we must see if the things that we were unhappy about were finally changing. Jenny and I agreed to go back and, over the course of a year, assess the situation. But by the spring of 1978 our minds were made up, and we had decided to apply for immigration papers to Canada.

The period of applying, being interviewed, being sent for a medical examination and waiting for an answer from the Canadian Embassy was a trying one, and we kept this all secret. We knew how negatively some of our friends and family would react to us "betraying" them and the country. In those days, to emigrate was still considered – by many Israelis – as letting the side down at the very least, if not as a downright act of betrayal. If immigrating to Israel is called *Aliyah* – going up – emigrating is called *Yeridah* – going down – and one who emigrates is labeled a *Yored* – one who has gone down, a word with a truly pejorative meaning. We were not only apprehensive about how our friends and family would react, but we also did not want to let our employer, the university, know until it was certain that we were leaving.

After we had filled out the application forms, had our interview at the Canadian Embassy, and undergone our medical examinations, I spent the last period of waiting, in the summer of 1978, in the middle of the Sinai desert doing my last ever stint of *miluim*.

There is an ironic twist to my final term in *miluim*, because it was so like being back as a national serviceman. When I reported for duty on the appointed day, I was processed by a very young clerk. "What's your serial number?" he barked.

I gave him my six-digit number.

"That's wrong," he said, officiously.

I repeated the same number and assured him it was correct. To this day, I can tell you what my serial number is.

"It can't be correct," he reproved me, "It only has six digits. You are missing a digit. All serial numbers have seven."

And then I understood.

"Not really," I said gently. "Way back in 1961, when I began my army service, there were only six digit numbers." He had the grace to laugh sheepishly.

I say that this last *miluim* was like coming full circle because, to my horror, I had been seconded to a national service unit and was to spend six never-ending weeks with them in the middle of the Sinai desert in the middle of summer. This was the first time that such a thing had ever happened to me, and it was dreadful. The people I was serving with were between the ages of 18 and 20, and we had absolutely no interests in common. After all, I was 34, had completed my studies, and was the father of three, our son Jonathan having been born in Edinburgh. Moreover, they had the true 'national service mentality,' and tried to use it to their advantage and my disadvantage. This meant that they would try and foist more than my share of duties, patrols and guards on me, the 'new kid,' thinking that I would not realize how I was being treated. I was not used to that kind of nastiness and trickery because it just never happened in a *miluim* unit, and it took me a few days to catch on to what was happening. When I did, I confronted the person in charge of drawing up the work, guarding and patrol rosters, and warned him that if he did not begin immediately to share the duties out fairly, I would see to it that he was put on a charge. That was the end of my troubles, but it was most unpleasant. And the rock music I had to live with for six whole weeks was sheer torture.

The news that we had been granted immigrant status to Canada came through that summer, while I was in *miluim*. In the first week of October, just after the historic visit of President Anwar Sadat of Egypt to Jerusalem, we left to seek a new life in Canada, once again immigrating to a country we had never even visited.

EPILOG

When I began to write this book I knew that, while it would touch in general terms on my life in Israel in the 1960s and 1970s, it would focus on the most formative aspect of that period – my active service in two wars and in *miluim* in *Tzahal*, The Defense Army of Israel, as a combat medic, a *chovesh kravi*. This was the one branch of the military profession with the aim of healing rather than destroying; I found that appealing.

Although, like many Israelis, I was reluctant and unenthusiastic about everything concerning the army, that does not in any way reflect on my feelings of love for Israel, or my deep-rooted conviction that every citizen's national obligation and privilege is to defend the country. I was never one of those who looked to *miluim* as a welcome break from the boring routine of civilian life, but simply accepted that military service was something all we Israelis without exception had to do, to be performed as faithfully and loyally as possible. And, despite my reluctance to serve in the army, to have fought in two of Israel's most important and critical wars is something of which I am proud. Actually, throughout all those years of service in a front line combat unit of *Tzahal*, I always described myself as a latent pacifist – in other words, I'd have loved to have been one, but my love for Israel and the understanding that military service was a collective national obligation overwhelmed such tendencies. In fact, I had no patience with the conscientious objectors (few though they were) of those days, seeing their behavior simply as a shirking of a solemn national duty resulting in someone else having to do the work, fight the battle and, possibly, die. Prior to the build-up to the Six Day War of 1967 thoughts such as these were entirely theoretical. But at some level of consciousness I knew that, if I were ever to be a full member of this society, I would have to do my share. And that is what I did, maybe reluctantly but always as faithfully and loyally as I could.

When I ran these thoughts past some Israeli friends, a few of them became almost indignant, saying things like, "All *Tzahal*'s soldiers are reluctant" – as if to imply, "What higher moral ground are *you* claiming for yourself by referring to yourself as a 'reluctant soldier'?" But, far from claiming any higher moral ground, I am not attempting to make any moral claims at all, being all too well aware that most of the soldiers serving in *Tzahal* feel much the same way that I do – that they have no alternative to doing what they do. This should never, however, be construed as enthusiasm for military service.

I have tried in this book to provide the most faithful description, without any embellishment, of my experiences, and then let them stand and speak for themselves, although I have for obvious reasons changed some of the names of people to avoid hurting anyone. The experiences I have described were not in any way unique. There are thousands of soldiers in *Tzahal* with stories just like mine; the only uniqueness of these stories is that they are *mine*, and that is why I have wanted to share them with you, my reader. In some ways I wish I could have avoided many of them, yet in some strange way I am proud to have had them. To no small extent they have shaped who I am.

Although we have visited Israel many times since leaving 25 years ago, like so many *Yordim* we have always had mixed feelings about our decision to emigrate. It is said that once you have lived in Israel, when you leave a part of yourself remains there. This is certainly true for Jenny and me.

About eight years ago, I was on a bus in Jerusalem and the man sitting opposite me looked very familiar. I lent over to him and asked him:

"Do you remember me?"

"No, sorry," he said.

"I was the medic who attended to your best friend when he was fatally wounded at the U.N. Headquarters on the second day of the Six Day War." It was my Yemenite comrade, and one of the ways I recognized him was that his clothes were spattered with paint spots – he was still painting houses. Although this was an emotionally charged encounter for me he was plainly not in the least moved by the experience, and so I muttered something like, "I now live in Canada. How are things for you?" And he replied with something noncommittal like, "Okay," and there the conversation ended. A few moments later the bus reached my stop, I got off, and never saw him again.

I returned to Jerusalem on sabbatical leave for six months beginning in September, 2001. This visit was at the height of the El Aksa (Second) Intifada, and morale was low. It was during this visit that I decided to write this book. In many ways the Israel of today, battling against ruthless suicide bombers, is a very different Israel from the one I've described in this book. But I believe that despite the appalling events and deeds that are being perpetrated, *Tzahal* remains a unique military force, one attempting against all odds to retain its moral standing.

There were several incidents that have moved me as I have been writing. One day I was taking a taxi to the Hebrew University on Mount Scopus and got chatting with the taxi driver. In the course of our conversation he told me where he had fought in the Six Day War – it turns out that we had been in the same battalion, and that we shared a number of army friends.

And then, on another occasion, I was going to a lecture at the Givat Ram campus of The Hebrew University and, having some time to spare, decided to look in at the Hebrew University High School next door, where I had been teaching at the time of the Six Day War. It was late afternoon, and there were just a few students around. I walked over to the Honor Board, and there were the names of all my ex-students and Nadav, who had died in the army. And then, to my shock and horror, I saw the name of a boy I had been particularly close to when I was his home room teacher – he, too, had been killed at some point, and I did not even know about it. But tragically that is the reality of Israel.

While in Jerusalem I decided to try and find Dudu, my company commander from the Six Day War. I knew that he had lived there at one time, and I found someone with that name in the telephone directory. With some trepidation I called and left a message, asking the person who answered to that name to call me back. Within a day, Dudu had called – and it was the *right* Dudu! I invited him out for coffee, and the following week we met at his favorite coffee shop. I was excited but also anxious about this meeting, because I didn't really know personally the Dudu that I so admired and, what is more, twenty-seven years had elapsed since I'd last seen him in Africa. Moreover, I was not sure how he would respond to the fact that I had emigrated.

I made a point of getting there early, and then at the appointed time a white haired, gentle looking man of 69 walked into the café, and the moment I saw his steely blue eyes I knew it was him. We spent a full two hours reminiscing. He did not remember all the incidents I have related in this book – after all, I was but one soldier in a company of around 100 in 1967, and one in a battalion of close to 1000 in 1973-4. But the more we spoke, the more he recalled. When I told him the story of the punishment he had given to the soldier in 1967 who came back from leave a day late, and how I had been chosen to go and speak to him and appeal to him to show leniency, he listened to me with the

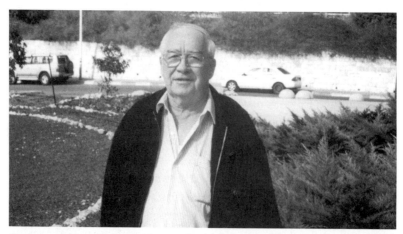

Dudu, my beloved commander, to whom I have dedicated this book. Jerusalem, 2002.

same look of caring attention that has always been his trademark. And when I had finished, ending by recounting how he had indeed altered the punishment, his response was true Dudu – he looked at me and said with a wry smile, "I'm glad I had the sense to listen to you." What a great response! He then recounted another story from the time he was an officer in another unit before joining our company in 1966; in this story, again, he had changed his mind about punishing a soldier who had refused the order to fire his rifle into the air to scare the people in a certain village. The care and thought that went into both of these decisions are precisely what makes him such a great man and such an outstanding leader. He also told me that he goes to the United Nations Headquarters in Jerusalem every Remembrance Day – the day prior to Israel's Independence Day, on which Israel remembers those who fell in its wars. He told me how he makes a speech to school children from the area at the ceremony at the memorial every year. The theme of his speech is always the same – "I tell them about incidents that show how special *Tzahal* is."

When we were about to leave, I looked at him across the table and said directly to him something I have never said directly to anyone before or since: "Dudu, you have no idea how much I admire you!" He was embarrassed but also, I believe, touched.

When our son and niece visited us in Jerusalem in the November of my sabbatical leave I took them to the United Nations Headquarters in order to show them where I had fought in the Six Day War and to describe the battle to them. The area at the entrance to the United Nations compound has been developed into a handsome boardwalk, the Tayelet, that stretches from Abu Tor in the north through the valley to the U.N. building in the south. On previous visits this spot was always teeming with tourists taking in the breathtaking views of the Old City of Jerusalem and the Judean Desert. There was a café right there that was invariably packed with people, and a throng of ice cream vending vans always did a roaring trade in the parking lot. Now, due to the Intifada, this magnificent location is deserted, and has regained something of the desolation and eeriness I associated with it from the Six Day War. A couple of people had been attacked by terrorists on the Tayelet in the preceding months, and the café had been burned down and looted. Three months later, at the beginning of February, a young woman was stabbed to death by terrorists on that same Tayelet.

There is a description of the battle that I took part in on a plaque on the Tayelet, and it explicitly mentions Battalion 161 – my battalion. As we read it out loud that late autumn day, I found myself asking: "Was that really me?" But then we walked across the parking lot to the memorial to the soldiers who fell on that day, and my question became immediately redundant. There were the names of the friends and comrades I had treated: Shimon, Yossie, Efraim and far too many others. It all came flooding back to me, but in its wake came another question: "Would you do it all again?" And my answer to this question is a clear and unequivocal one: "Yes, terrible though it was, I would!"

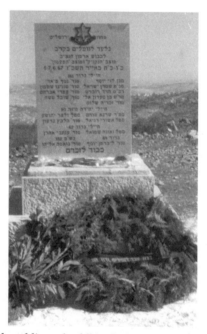

War memorial to the soldiers who fell in the battle for the U.N. Headquarters in June, 1967.